FIGHTING FIERCELY:
Unveiling the Unknown about Endometriosis

A guide for educating, enlightening,
and empowering women and their loved ones.

Michelle N. Johnson, LMT CIMI

DEDICATION

This book is dedicated to every little girl that is being told right now that the debilitating pain she feels is merely a rite of passage into womanhood. This book is dedicated to every woman who has ever been told, in-spite-of: physical, mental, and emotional evidence that nothing is wrong with her, only to be later diagnosed with varying stages of Endometriosis. It is my hope that every woman reading this will be equipped with the knowledge and awareness to avoid the commonplace delay of eight to ten years between symptom and diagnosis. In addition, this book is dedicated to every woman who has ever been ignored, dismissed, or made to feel inferior by those in the medical community because of the ignorance surrounding the subject of Endometriosis. This book is dedicated to every woman who feels like there is no one who understands her, because, they don't understand Endometriosis. This book is dedicated to every woman who feels that she doesn't have a voice to make decisions regarding her treatment of Endometriosis. This book is dedicated to all of my Endo Sisters - the more than 176 million women, teens, and young girls worldwide, affected by this disease every day.

KEEP FIGHTING!

DISCLAIMER

I am NOT a medical doctor. Nor, am I an expert in diagnosing or treating Endometriosis. The message conveyed in this book is based on my own personal experiences with battling endometriosis, and therefore, this book should be used for informational and educational purposes only. Nothing in this book should be taken as medical expertise or advice. It is not intended to be a substitute or replacement for professional medical treatment and care. If you suspect that you may have Endometriosis, or if you have been medically diagnosed with Endometriosis, please consult your primary care practitioner.

CONTENTS

ACKNOWLEDGMENTS

I have to give an incredibly special and heartfelt "thank you" to one of my dearest and closest friends, Ayana Evans. I thank you for planting the seed for this book four years ago, by telling me that my story needed to be told, and that many women would find triumph in the transparency of my truth. (Even though I told you, "there was no way in hell I was letting anybody all up in my bid'ness like that!").

I would also like to thank my parents. To my mother, Dorse Kelly, I forever thank you for continually praying "without ceasing" for your daughter. There is nothing that can withstand the power of a Praying Mother! I would also like to thank my Father, Hayward Johnson Jr., I thank you for always listening and for always picking up the phone (no matter the time, day or night). I thank God for choosing you to be my parents and I could not have picked a better pair myself. I love you both to life!

To my: friends, nutrition coaches, and life style re-arrangers Marquese Martin-Hayes and Olivia Gomez-you guys have literally changed my life! There will never be enough words to express my gratitude!

To my writing coach, Erika *The Unstoppable Woman* Gilchrist, thank you for giving me "The Blueprint." Your foundation helped me to take my vision from brain to book. There are not too many people who can *read* me as well as you.

To my phenomenal editor, Christine Weatherby – one word – AMAZING! I am forever grateful for the Divine Connection that brought you into my life.

To my graphic designer Sandra Ballenger: Thank you for your patience, your diligence, and your unwavering commitment to making sure every piece of this project was absolutely perfect!

To all of my Courageous Conquerors and Bossette Mastermind Sisters; Infinite thanks for: all of the words of encouragement, motivation, and accountability.

To my CCM Coach Da-Nay Macklin, I thank you for believing in me when I couldn't see far enough to believe in myself. Thank you for fanning the flames every time I thought my fire was about to go out!

To my *ride- it- to- the- wheels- fall-off -there- through- everything big sistah-friend* Lanise R. Washington: Thank you for calling and texting me every day in that final week to make sure that I stayed on track, kept focused, stayed off Facebook, and got it done!

To my amazing *Endo Sisters* and support groups: I thank you for understanding in the way that nobody else can understand.

Most of all, I thank my Heavenly Father for trusting me to be His vessel in delivering this message of advocacy and awareness. I pray that everyone who reads this book will be ministered to in a particularly tangible and meaningful way.

There was once a time when I cried out in frustration:

"Dear Lord, Why Me?!"

Today I stand with a Spirit of willingness and cooperation, saying

"Here I am Lord, Use Me!"

FORWARD

By: Celeste Parker, Author

Cold cures are common, for Endo there isn't
Red spots look back from wherever you're sittin'
Brown paper bags that hide tampons with strings
These are a few of our feminine things
Prescription phonies, nurses note, doctors doodle
3rd degrees, surgeries, kit and caboodle
Wild guesses tried, maxi pads that have wings
These are a few of our feminine things
Girls in white dresses get the blues if "she" crashes
Down the hall, bathroom stall into she dashes
It feels like summer, hot flashes she brings
These are a few of our feminine things

The sounds of girlhood aren't...so...honest. That is, until Michelle Johnson answered the call and pulled the alarm. With wit, raw realness and analogies that no longer acquiesce, but answer the questions of both genders, Johnson lays down sticks and stones and packs a powerful punch with her words of wisdom about Endometriosis. From dispelling the myth about passing the painful baton of bleeding being our birthright, to discussions as intimate as how to tell Mr. Right that you feel like you have nothing left-Johnson's strength sticks, her passion moves. Her expertise makes her a woman worth knowing, while her emotional experience embraces you like one of the girls. No longer killing our spirits softly, with each page she equips us to instead face the opponent (Endo), put on our own gloves, come out swinging and live a healthy, whole, victorious life.

When it hurts—fight! Ever fiercely!
Give it all you have
Remember you have it
It doesn't have you
And then you won't feel so bad

Celeste T. Parker, Stage 4 Endometriosis Survivor
Author, *Pigs Don't Wear Pearls* Children's Books
www.pigsdontwearpearls.com

PROLOUGE:

1987, Age 11

Giving myself the once over in the bathroom mirror, I decided that I was looking pretty cute. Although I would rather be wearing jeans, this white lace dress isn't too bad. Although mama could've got me some better looking shoes, it will still be okay, because, they won't see them in the picture. I do love my hair though, and I'm not sure if it's nervousness or excitement, but my stomach is starting to feel really weird. I know I'm not hungry because I just finished eating. Maybe I'm just really "geeked" to get to school and see what the other girls are going to be wearing. Dang... I am really starting to feel sick, like I need to throw up or something. Maybe I should try to go to the bathroom before I leave. The last thing I need is to be stuck in the bathroom at school, peeing when it's my turn to take my picture.....

As I made my way to the bathroom the butterflies that were jousting in my stomach had started to get worse. For a very brief moment, I thought, maybe I was getting my period... but nahhh it couldn't be... not now... not *today!* I had heard some of the older girls talk about getting their periods. Since I was only 11, I just knew I had at least another year or more before I got mine. Lord knows I was not looking forward to it at all! As I sat there on the toilet waiting for myself to finish, all of a sudden I started to panic. All of a sudden, it was like I knew, but I didn't want to know. In fact, I couldn't help but know. As I yanked the tissue off the roll and prepared to wipe myself, I took in a deep breath. I should have just dropped the tissue in the toilet, but I didn't; instead, I slowly brought the tissue in front of my face and there it was staring back at me.... the bright pink flush of dampness that would forever destroy my prepubescent, tomboyish life!

NO NO NO NO NO! This cannot be happening! Why God why? Why why why why why? Why? Why ME? why NOW? Why TODAY? Could this not have happened to me on a worse day! I am so not prepared for this! I am so not interested in this!!! Dang! Now I gotta call my mamma......

"Hey Ma."

"Hey girl, why haven't you left for school yet?"

"It happened ma."

"What happened girl? What are you talking about?"

"You knoooooow, 'it'."

"It? Girl, if you don't speak up - You know I'm at work!"

"Maaaa you KNOOOWW, 'IT'… (In a hushed whisper) my period!"

When my mother burst out into uncontrollable laughter, I did not find it at all amusing.

"Don't laugh mama. This is NOT funny. It is not funny at all…."

As my mother proceeded to talk me through what I needed to do in order to "get myself together", the rest of my day immediately filled with dread. In fact, I no longer cared about the stupid pictures anymore. When they finally called my name to step up to the podium and have my pictures taken, all I could hear, feel, or think about was the pain in my stomach pounding away like a bass drum. I thought that I would pass out at any moment. Thankfully, I didn't. As I stood there posing with the biggest, brightest, smile I could muster, the only thing I could think about was: *"I have to deal with this sh*t for the next how many years?"*

1988, Age 12

I really wish mama would have let me stay home from school today, but I knew she wouldn't, especially with today being the day for us to take the Constitution Test. If we don't pass this test, we don't graduate and my mama is not having that! But I am cramping so bad I can barely focus on the words that are in front of me. Maybe if I just get through the test then she'll let me come home from school early. I swear, I think I'm about to die! I was cramping so bad this morning when I got up that I could hardly walk. And now sitting here, I'm so doggone dizzy I feel like I'm on a roller coaster ride at Great America. Man, I have a headache out-of-this world! And at this point I could not give a damn about the three branches of government or who gets to veto a bill in Congress! All I want to do is go home and lay down. This period crap is for the birds! I thought it was supposed to get easier as time went on ... but it's been over a year and it is not getting any better...Oh my God what the heck is going on? My head is pounding, the room is spinning, it won't slow down, and the room is getting dark...

It was not until I woke up in the principal's office, staring into my Daddy's eyes, that I realized that I had passed out in class. While it was true that I had wanted to stay home from school, this was not the way I had planned getting early dismissal from class! As we rode home with me curled up in the front seat of the car, I was in so much pain that I couldn't even speak. When my dad asked me what was wrong, all I could do was point to my stomach as he replied: *"Oh, women's troubles...Don't worry"*, he'd said, *"I'll get you to your auntie soon enough, and she'll be able to take care of you."*

My legs were all but dead weight by the time we made it home, and my dad had to practically carry me into the house. No sooner than I had reached the edge of the bed, I collapsed. That's when the pain really let loose! My aunt padded casually into the room with a steaming cup of Lipton tea and two of the biggest pills that I had ever seen in my life! As my dad excused himself, she sat softly on the edge of the bed and scooped me up in a warm, half- embrace. She broke the chalky white, egg-shaped pills in half and held the porcelain cup as I slowly sipped, "slurp....uggh." After gagging and spitting them up a couple of times, I finally got the pills down and continued sipping the tea. As my aunt, massaged tiny little circles around my stomach, she looked at me with a certain, finite surety. Plainly and calmly she had been assuring me that, *"this is all a part of being a woman, baby."*

*Well damn all that! If this is what being a woman is, y'all can KEEP that sh*t!*

Before my verbal protests could find their way to my lips, the pain pills had begun to take effect and I was well on my way to sleep... sweet sleep, and feeling no pain! At least, for the moment...

1992, age 16

Dayum! I do not have time for this today! I have got graduation practice first thing this morning and I am not trying to be late! I've already soaked through two pads   this morning and it's not even eight o'clock yet! I'm wearing the darkest jeans I could find and I've got about three more pads stacked together covering me from front to back, so, nothing will leak out! I feel like I'm wearing a diaper, but I'm still scared that I could just spill out at any minute. THIS SUCKS! I'm so tired I could probably lay down and sleep for three days straight, but graduation is just around the corner and I am not about to miss practice. If I can just get down the block to Nesha's house then maybe she'll let me crash for a few minutes! I have already taken three Advil and they are doing absolutely NOTHING to help!

"Heyyyyy girl, what's up?"

"Gurrrrrrl, you already know! Can I just lay down for minute before we head out?"

"Yeah, but we can't wait too long or else you know they'll start making those tardy calls."

"That's cool. I just need to rest a bit and give these cramps some time to settle down."

I laid there for what seemed like hours. By this point, my closest friends had already become familiar with my monthly routine, so, they were more than willing to step in and help me out, when needed. Always the incredibly supportive friend, KaNesha helped me get my "Period Pack" together which consisted of: an entire package of pads, a ½ bottle of *Tylenol,* wet wipes, and an extra pair of panties (just in case). As always, KaNesha helped me find a way to store it discreetly in my backpack, and then, we were on our way. It was the end of the school year. It was my senior year, and I had a graduation to practice for…

CHAPTER 1
W....T...F?!

"This is some buuullllsh*t!" ~Bernie Mac.

November 2007

I had always had "heavy periods", but *this* was something completely and entirely different! After 20+ years of going through the pain, the cramps, the swollen breasts, and utter fatigue month-after-month, you would think I would have it down by now. But something strange was definitely going on this time. At first I didn't think too much of it; I just figured it was stress. After all, it had been just about a year since I quit my "good job" to follow my faith into the land of entrepreneurship by staring my new career as a licensed massage therapist and corporate wellness consultant. Shortly after that, new management had taken over the apartment building where I had been living for the past ten years, causing me to have to move rather suddenly. Luckily, a great apartment opened up just two buildings over, so the move was relatively quick and painless.

In the meantime, my business had accelerated and I was now doing very well financially! In fact, *Essential~E Therapeutic Massage & Bodywork* had just secured our first major corporate wellness client and I was actually starting to look into hiring my very first employee! With all these major changes happening so close together, I just figured my body was overreacting and would settle down as soon as I did. So, when the bleeding got heavier, I doubled up on the *Always* pads and pressed forward. When the cramps intensified, I doubled up on the *Aleeve* and emotionally pushed through the pain. When the lethargy and fatigue set in, I shook it off. I did not have time to worry about myself. I had: a wellness program to implement, a new business to dig into, prospective candidates to interview, and a new deluxe studio apartment overlooking lake Michigan to decorate. I had book club hosting duties in December and an upcoming summer mission trip to Kenya, Africa teaching infant massage to mothers! I did not have time to be sidetracked by impending health problems!

As symptoms continued, I had no choice but to listen to the changes in my body when the time in between my periods had begun to get shorter, first every 28, then 21, and finally, about every 14 days. However, I kept telling myself that as soon as everything slowed down, eventually, I would too. As a grown woman, embarrassing doesn't begin to describe the anguish I felt the first time I bled through my clothes while I was at work. I had not had to deal with such mishaps since the first few months of starting my period. Thankfully, I was able to clean myself up and hide the damage before anyone else *spotted* the mishap.

I found myself going through multiple 28-packs of pads originally designed for extra heavy and overnight flow in a matter of days. I mastered the art of discreetly layering sheets of newspaper between myself and the seats of my friends' car when we went out "kicking it…" just in case. Eventually, all the over the counter pain meds stopped working, and it started to feel like a fleet of thoroughbreds were tap-dancing across my lower back. I became frighteningly alarmed when I started passing blood clots that were: as thick and solid as a fist, black, and opaque as ink. Thanks to *Web MD*,[1] I was convinced I had found the answer to my troubles following a self-diagnosis of PMDD (Pre Menstrual Dysphoric Disorder).

I continued to reason with myself that all I needed to do was to complete my current to-do list, make it through all of the forthcoming holiday festivities, and then I would be fine. If something were actually proven to be the matter, I thought I would have adequate time to heal and recuperate, because, I always took the first week of the new year off. So, I rationalized that all I needed to do was make it to the new year. Now was not the time to slow down! I was just getting started…..besides, wasn't this, *"just all a part of being a woman?"*

Saturday, February 23, 2008

Boy oh boy…the ways your life can change within the span of a month! It feels like much longer since last we spoke, but a lifetime of things have changed since[then]. At first I was going on-and-on about how 2008 was shaping up to be a great year and 'bout how I was meeting some pretty cool people…that was around the

18th of January…right around the time I THOUGHT I was catching the flu. I started off lethargic and feverish(slightly) and somewhat crampy. But, I chalked it up to the crazy fluctuation of 50 degree to minus 3degree winter days. So, I stocked up on all my Advil, Tylenol, Nyquil, Alka-Seltzer, Theraflu, and the like. By Sunday the 20th, it was really starting to set in, so I figured [it was running its course, and] I'd be good to go by at least Tuesday. No such luck! By Tuesday, my [continued] temp of 103 was pushing strong and by Wednesday the cramping in my lower left side was becoming unbearable. By Thursday morning, I was on the phone with the doctor and by Friday, the 25th, I was on my way to the emergency room with 'suspected diverticulitis' that was on the verge of rupture [either that or a burst appendix: they weren't really sure]. Well, after calling my mom, and dad and getting over there, thus began the testing frenzy and about nine hours later I was admitted to the hospital!

It would still be another couple of days of 'suspected this', and 'preliminary signs of that', until the final diagnosis was made: severe [stage 4]'endometriosis' in the left fallopian tube and ovary with a 'hydrosalpinx' in my right. Basically, there was fluid buildup in my tubes which apparently caused massive amounts of inflammation and swelling. The swelling was so bad that, that this stupid 'chocolate cyst' was pressing against my ureter, causing a backup of urine and potential infection of my kidney. This meant that over the course of the next few days, that I would have to have a tube inserted in my kidneys to drain out the excess urine to avoid continued infection. So, now, I got that stupid piss bag hooked up to me making me feel like I'm 172 years old. Apparently they went and drained some of the fluid outta my fallopian tube [and did some biopsies] to confirm that it is this endometriosis! And of course the wonderful joy of being poked and prodded every which way from Sunday. I know right ! Yeeeaaahhh ME – big fun right! I finally got to come home on the 28th after having a stint place inside my bladder (thank God,) so that I can at least attempt to pee normally.

I have been set up for a hormone/pain relief/surgery protocol that is planned to be carried out over the next 6-8 weeks!

To say that those ten days back in January 2008 would forever change my life would probably be the grossest understatement ever uttered by anyone on this side of God's green earth! The panic, uncertainty, bewilderment, utter confusion, and fear that gripped me during that nine hour interrogation of just about every open cavity and orifice in my body was unlike anything I've ever experienced before or since. While many of the details of that narcotic/antibiotic induced haze at times escape me, I do vividly remember the numerous rounds of blood draws and injections. I candidly recall the names of drugs such as *Dilaudid* and *Fentanyl* being tossed around as I made several trips back and forth to exam and procedure rooms for various ultrasounds, MRI's, and a myriad of scopes.

One of the most traumatizing memories I still have of that time is waiting for my parents to arrive thinking wearily to myself *"Oh MY God, I'm going to die! Right here, in this messy emergency room, without my mamma and daddy, with all my ass and 'cooch' hanging out for all the world to see! And the worst part is, no one can even tell me what the f*ck is wrong with me!"*

Even after being admitted into the hospital, it still took another three days and an entire team of doctors to actually figure out "what was wrong with me." The diagnosis finally came after, basically, eliminating a list of diseases that I *didn't* have. Meanwhile, the doctors had continued to scare me sh*tless in the process! On many occasions the doctors were talking around me as if I wasn't even in the room. They used words like: *HIV, ovarian/cervical cancer, damaged, no children, worst case we've ever seen, ruptured tubes,* and *hysterectomy* with such brandished about casualty that I couldn't tell if they were attempting diagnoses or ordering lunch!

Hearing the words *cancer* and *hysterectomy*, for me, a 30-something, single, African American woman with no children, were tantamount to a death sentence. An avalanche of tears billowed down my cheeks as my soul simultaneously took flight through my silent, grief stricken gasp! My hospital room instantaneously morphed into an episode of the old Charlie Brown cartoon, and the chief "specialist" on my "case" had become Charlie's teacher, because the only thing I remembered hearing after that was *'wah wah wah wah wah wahhhhh...'*

When the verdict finally came, Stage 4 Endometriosis- sometimes called *Endo* for short- I still wasn't entirely clear as to what exactly that meant. Before this diagnosis the only *"Endo"* I knew anything about was courtesy of *Dr. Dre, Snoop Dogg, & Tha Dogg Pound!* Therefore, I patiently tried to absorb the doctor's attempt at an explanation about randomly displaced uterine lining floating to areas outside of the uterus, and the subsequent results thereof. In between my blank stares and rapidly repeated blinking, I couldn't help but briefly smirk when I thought to myself, *'Endo.... what tha f*ck is she talkin' bout! Am I s'posed to put five on this sh*t or what?'*

All I knew was that after looking at my biopsy results, the doctors had concluded that I'd had this disease for at **least** ten years. Furthermore, my case was so severe, and my tumor so large, that the entire left side of my reproductive system (ovaries and fallopian tube), would have to be completely removed along with several smaller cysts from the right side. The doctors told me that having surgery was the best course of treatment advisable at this stage, and depending on my "family planning" options, I might want to consider having a complete hysterectomy.

After basically telling them to go f*ck themselves at the suggestion of a full hysterectomy, *(I wasn't even about to entertain that option, I was still trying to wrap my brain around the concept of this 'Endo' and this surgery I would inevitably have to have)* I was then told that following a successful surgery, when the time came, that while I *could* still get pregnant, I would likely have many complications and would probably be considered high risk from the onset. At this point, who had time to think about getting pregnant? I wasn't even dating anyone! All I wanted was to stop this bleeding, schedule this surgery, yank whatever the f*ck it was that was destroying my insides OUT, and get on about the business of getting back to normal. Little did I realize, that my current sense of normalcy was lost. I wondered if I would ever find my normal again?

The day before being released, I was given a plan for the follow up care leading to my surgery scheduled for March 2008. Because of the massive amount of blood loss over the past several months, I had become severely anemic. Normal hemoglobin levels for women are around "12 to 16 gm/dL [gram per deciliter of

5

whole blood]" [2] In contrast, my levels were hovering somewhere around a 6 at the time, so it was necessary to place me on an iron supplement, *Repliva,* in order to replenish my hemoglobin levels. Otherwise, there would be an increased risk that I would need a blood transfusion during the surgery. No way in hell was I risking that! It was literally a miracle that I was able to even stand, let alone walk and move. At least now I had a real explanation for why I'd been run down for the past three months and it had not been the *Chicago Hawk!*

In addition to the iron pills, I was to begin a six month round of a drug called *Lupron®,* which I was supposed to get via injection starting that night, and continuing once a month, until three months after my surgery. The reason I needed this drug, as explained to me at the time, was to stop the tumor (e.g. chocolate cyst) growth and potentially even shrink it. The doctors needed it to get down to a "safely operable" size. As long as I had my period, the tumor risked continued growth. Doctor's theorized that if we could stop my period, we would stop the growth; so, they essentially used this drug to put my body into a "chemically induced state of menopause" (yes you heard me -MENOPAUSE) at 33 years old!

By this time I was so overwhelmed and inundated with information, I pretty much thought, *yeah, yeah, okay, whatever…if it will help, just give it to me and let me go!* In addition to the *Lupron®,* I was also prescribed *Danazol,* a hormonal "add-back" medication, *(WTF is an add back and why do I need it?),* along with *Mefenamic (meff-en-AM-ick) Acid,* to help control the pain and the bleeding. I was to report back for a follow up appointment in a few days. And that was that! So, with a "plan" in place, a stint in my kidney, four different drugs, and a ton of brochures and pamphlets, I was off to prepare for surgery and to adjust to my life with this newly diagnosed disease.

After returning home, I sat on my living room sofa, emptily glancing down at all the *stuff* in my lap. I tried to recall all of the explanations, information, policies, procedures, timelines, instructions, reasons, and rationales undeservedly thrust upon me over the past few days. By now, my mind was swimming in a vast sea of both confusion and contempt. One thing was abundantly and incredibly clear: I had heard the words, read the brochures, seen the diagrams, talked to the doctors, asked my questions, and taken my notes (in typical Virgo fashion), and had been diagnosed with Endometriosis! In contrast, I still had no tangible, meaningful, unequivocal idea as to what any of this actually meant. I was still pretty clueless, and very much in a state of W.....T.....F!?

CHAPTER 2
ENDO EXPLAINED

"Upside down...boy ya turn me, inside out, and round and round..."
~Diana Ross.

Yeah, I know. If you're anything like me, just reading through that has probably sent you into a cranial tailspin! Imagine how I felt living through it!?

Endometriosis.org[3] and *The Endometriosis Association*[4] were the first websites that I found that helped to give me my first sense of clarity. In fact, the information that I found there helped me to wrap my mind and my emotions around the levity and the magnitude of what I was facing. The information magnified my sense of understanding as to how my life would forever be changed. Since then I have found many other incredible resources, that have not only helped me, but have also helped the more than 176 million women who are affected by this disease.

Because these resources were (and are) so incredibly helpful to me, I just wanted to share some of what I gleaned from a few of them in order to help educate, enlighten, and empower you to plainly understand and to better make sense of your own journey battling this disease. These websites/resources are also helpful if you have a spouse, significant other, mother, sister, daughter, or loved one who is also living this experience. They will also be incredibly useful in helping you understand many of the multi-syllabic and brain-warping words, terms, and phrases, that you're likely to encounter as you continue to read this book!

When I was released following my initial hospital visit, I knew it would be close to two months before I would have to go back in for surgery. In the meantime, I was determined not to let this new "protocol" get to me; therefore, I tried to return to business as usual. I started on my new meds and began interviewing potential employees for my business. I returned to my part-time job as a massage therapist and continued working diligently to fulfill my goal of starting my own practice.

...Everyone was welcoming me back, asking, "how it was going." Even Carlos asked me how I felt about the information that the doctors had given me. At first, I was like yeah, sure, it's okay. I'm pretty confident [although I really wasn't]. Then he said, "That's good , but always do outside research for yourself – just to be sure..." I had never thought to look any further than the information I'd initially been given. Like so many newly diagnosed Endo Women, I had taken the doctor's words as law, even though much of what I'd been told was very unsettling to me. In contrast, Carlo's words stayed with me, and when I went home that evening I began to scour the internet, searching for all things Endometriosis. And then I found this awesome website, endometriosis.org, – and I'm so glad I did! All the information mimicked everything the doctor's had said, but to an infinite degree of detail. There was information all about: the surgery, the meds, the treatment options, how the meds actually worked in your body, step-by-step information of the surgical procedures, post-op care, pre-op care, and more! I was really nervous and apprehensive about things before, especially knowing I'd be in there (surgery) for up to five hours. Now, after visiting that site I was like Ahhhhhhh – EXHALE.

As I mentioned in Chapter One, when my diagnosis was finally given a name "Endometriosis", I was completely and utterly clueless as to what this even meant. I had no idea that cases of this disease could be traced back several decades, with one of the earliest cases being mentioned as far back as 1860.[5] I thought this was some new phenomenon, unique to me. I had no idea that it affected a number of celebrities, entrepreneurs, and business women, many of whom I looked up to and admired, including: Whoopi Goldberg, Hillary Clinton, Susan Sarandon, Cindy Lauper, Marilyn Monroe, Tia Mowry, even Queen Victoria. [6]

When my friend first mentioned to me that it was probably a good idea to do my own homework, in addition to the information I'd been given from the doctors, something struck in me. Thinking back on it now, I'm pretty sure I was simply too overwhelmed at the time to have thought of it myself. However, when I heard him say it, the textbook Virgo, researcher, and information gatherer that I am was ignited. I was determined to educate myself as much as possible in the next two months before going back "under the knife" for surgery.

The following information is just a small glimpse into the vast amount of what is available regarding Endometriosis. This particular material was especially helpful in guiding me in understanding the definition, symptoms, and treatment options at my disposal. You may find that the discussion of these three particular topics will bring you more clarity with your own informational research.

What *is Endometriosis?*
According to their website, **The Endometriosis Association** (2014) defines Endometriosis as:

> A painful, chronic disease that affects at least 6.3 million women and girls in the U.S., 1 million in Canada, and millions more worldwide. It occurs when tissue like that which lines the uterus (tissue called the endometrium) is found outside the uterus -- usually in the abdomen on the ovaries, fallopian tubes, and ligaments that support the uterus; the area between the vagina and rectum; the outer surface of the uterus; and the lining of the pelvic cavity. Other sites for these endometrial growths may include the bladder, bowel, vagina, cervix, vulva, and in abdominal surgical scars. Less commonly they are found in the lung, arm, thigh, and other locations.

> This misplaced tissue develops into growths or lesions which respond to the menstrual cycle in the same way that the tissue of the uterine lining does: each month the tissue builds up, breaks down, and sheds. Menstrual blood flows from the uterus and out of the body through the vagina, but the blood and tissue shed from endometrial growths has no way of leaving the body. This results in internal bleeding, breakdown of the blood and tissue from the lesions, and inflammation -- and can cause pain, infertility, scar tissue formation, adhesions, and bowel problems. [7]

Once I fully understood what this disease was and how it "worked", all of the symptoms that I had experienced over the past year made complete sense to me. I also had a more vivid and thorough comprehension of what was happening to the inside of my body, as well as, on the outside. The brochure "What is

Endometriosis" (2010) by the Endometriosis Association explained: Sometimes, these tissues develop into what are called 'nodules, 'tumors', 'lesions', 'implants', or 'growths'. [8] Additionally, I found out:

> They are also commonly referred to as endometriomas, or chocolate cysts which get their name "from the dark old blood that grossly resembles chocolate…Most women will get them in the ovary on the left side of the body… Usually, the size of an endometrioma ranges from about half an inch (grape size) to four inches or more (softball size) in diameter. [9]

As it turned out, my case of Endo was very similar to the example mentioned here. Not only was my "chocolate cyst" located on my left ovary, but the disease had so viciously ravaged not only my ovary, but also my left fallopian tube and the surrounding structures, that the entire left side of my reproductive system had to be removed. This heartbreaking outcome would significantly reduce my options for having children in the future. And while most cysts range from one to four inches in diameter, mine was almost larger than six inches! This was the reason for the intense pain on the left side of my body that was causing the disruption to the proper function of my urinary system.

Symptoms

> One of the biggest problems with treating Endometriosis is obtaining an early, accurate diagnosis. In many cases there can be as much as an 8.5 year delay between initial symptom onset and a final diagnosis. [10]

As I mentioned earlier, when my definitive results came back, I was told that based on the severity of the disease present in my body (also referenced as one of the *"worst cases"* they'd ever seen), it was plausible to conclude that I'd been suffering with the disease for at least ten years! *At least*, meaning here is a very strong possibility that I may have had it for even longer!

In the prologue, I described how my first debilitating experience with painful periods, at the tender age of 12, caused me to lose consciousness. The incident was met very tenderly, albeit it nonchalantly, with the grand declaration of the so called fact that what I was experiencing, horrendous as it was, should have been heralded as a welcoming badge of honor. According to my elders, I should have been celebrating my inauguration into the realm of biological womanhood. Unfortunately, too many of our Endo Sisters are frivolously dismissed in much the same way by many well-intentioned, though grossly unaware: parents, spouses, family, friends, and most dishearteningly, medical professionals.

Many women with Endometriosis may experience a monthly hell of symptoms that reach far beyond the typical bloating, cramping, and physical discomforts that often accompany a woman's menstrual cycle. Some of the more significant signs/symptoms of Endometriosis, as described by the U.S. National Library of Medicine (2011), are:

> ...Very strong pains and cramps in the lower abdomen. To start off with, these normally occur during the woman's monthly period, but as the illness progresses they may be felt at other times of the month too. The pain sometimes radiates to the woman's back and down her legs, and is often associated with nausea, vomiting and diarrhea. [11]

Figure 1:

The following symptoms may[also]be signs of Endometriosis...

- Strong period pains (dysmenorrhea) that are so bad that low doses of painkillers do not help and the affected women are unable to perform their daily activities or go to work.

- Pain during sexual intercourse (dyspareunia) or afterwards, which is normally described as burning or cramp-like.

- Pain of varying intensity in different parts of the lower abdomen that also occurs between periods. [12]

Figure 2:

Additional symptoms,

as noted by the U.S. National Library of Medicine (2011) may include: diarrhea or constipation (in particular in connection with menstruation).

Some women may also experience:

- Abdominal bloating (in particular in connection with menstruation)
- Heavy or irregular bleeding
- Fatigue [13]

Figure 3:

While Endo associated pain can occur anytime it may be felt most often...

- Before/during/after menstruation
- During ovulation
- In the bowel during menstruation
- When passing urine
- During or after sexual intercourse
- In the lower back region [14]

It is important to interject that, experiencing any one or more of these symptoms at any given time, does not definitively indicate that you have Endometriosis. However, if you have continually experienced several of these symptoms, often in conjunction with one another over a prolonged period of time, then you may want to consider discussing the possibility of a diagnosis with you doctor.

In deciding whether or not to discuss Endo with your doctor, it is also necessary to be mindful that you could have Endometriosis even if you fail to show all of the symptoms. According to Institute for Quality and Efficiency in Health Care (October 2011):

> Not all women who have endometriosis experience noticeable symptoms. Those who do not have symptoms often do not notice changes in the lower abdomen at all. For this reason it is difficult to estimate how many women actually have endometriosis. It is believed that about 40 to 60 out of 100 women (40% to 60%) who suffer from very painful periods have endometriosis. Endometriosis can either be mild (stages I and II) or moderate to severe (stages III and IV). Women who have moderate or severe endometriosis often have problems getting pregnant, particularly if their ovaries and fallopian tubes are affected. Mild endometriosis usually does not affect fertility. [15]

Of all the symptoms associated with Endometriosis, one of the scariest and most impactful is infertility. "It is estimated that 30-40% of women with Endometriosis are sub-fertile." [16] Whereas the thought of Endo associated infertility can be quite daunting, the positive side to this statistic is that, more than half of women affected with Endo (60%) can be successful with carrying one or more healthy pregnancies to term!

Aside from the symptoms already mentioned, my experiences also included: extended periods of bleeding (no pun intended) that would last anywhere from 10 to over 30 days, consecutively! I'm talking full on flow, pouring out like water, filling up the longest, biggest *Always* pad ever made (14-15 inches front to back) in a matter of hours. The bleeding would continue repeatedly, day-after-day, for weeks at a time! Not to mention the copious amount of blood clots that would fill the toilet every time I went to pee! If you were to close your eyes and stand outside the bathroom, you would think I had diarrhea from the sound of it, but it was actually the rapid passing of multiple blood clots!

One time in particular, I thought I had to be having a miscarriage, even though I'd been sexually abstinent for nearly three years. I remember, a sharp shooting pain sent me running to the bathroom, and upon pulling down my panties, it looked as if someone had just dumped a large jar of grape jelly in them! Blood clots were literally spilling over from my panties onto the floor! I screamed so loudly I scared myself! I sat there for a moment on the toilet, poking and sniffing, and examining them, trying to figure out if any of my organs had fallen out! The smell of iron in the air was so strong, it instantly made me nauseous! I remember having to scoop the clots out of my underwear before I could even begin to clean myself up! I was horrified!

By the time I managed to get to the shower it appeared that the bleeding finally started to subside. As I stepped out and started to lightly dry myself, I thought nothing of the residual moisture trickling down my legs. I often liked to air dry after showering; so, I paid no mind to being naked as I shuffled my way from my bathroom to the closet to get a fresh set of pajamas. When I turned around to head back, I nearly tripped over my own feet! There, highlighting my short walk from room-to-room, was a crimson trail of blood, littered with more clots, culminating in a small puddle in front of my nightstand. Panicked, I shoved the pajamas in between my legs and ran back to the backroom, trying frantically to clean myself (again). I threw the pajamas in the sink and turned on the cold water to flush away the blood before any stains set in. I hurried to clean the floor and put on a clean set of undies and a pad, before the next rush of bloodiness came gushing out!

I can't tell you if it was the fear, the frustration, the unexpectedness or the flat out grossness of it all that sent me over the edge.... but that night, when I finally hoisted my aching self into bed all I could do was cry! There was nothing to help me: no doctor, no website, no pamphlet, no *YouTube* video, nothing...nothing, nothing, nothing - that could have prepared me for that sh*t!

Ladies, if you are reading this, and if this parallels anything remotely close to any experience you've had, please hear me - loud and clear - when I tell you: THIS IS NOT NORMAL! And anyone that tells you it is, is lying either to you, or to themselves!

Diagnosis

One of the primary reasons that it is often difficult to accurately diagnose Endometriosis is because many of the symptoms often mimic those of other similar reproductive disorders. Fibroids, Pelvic Inflammatory Disease (PID), Pre Menstrual Dysphoric Disorder (PMDD), ovarian cysts, irritable bowel syndrome, ovarian cancer, appendicitis, and ectopic pregnancies can all have symptoms similar to those experienced with Endo. [17]

In my own journey, when I noticed a marked change in my symptoms, I initially thought I had PMDD, defined by Mary M. Gallenberg, MD as: "...a severe, sometimes disabling extension of premenstrual syndrome (PMS). PMDD causes extreme mood shifts that can disrupt your work and damage your relationships." [18]

It wasn't until I was in the hospital, in crisis mode, undergoing several simultaneous tests, scans, and biopsies, that I was definitively and accurately diagnosed. As I was laying there, I thought about my own history, and it dawned on me that, over the years, there were many abnormalities that might have signaled earlier stages of Endo. For example, I had: abnormal pap smears, ovarian and uterine cysts/polyps, and pre-cancerous growths on my cervix. I wondered why I had never been tested for Endo, or why the possibility had never even been considered by previous medical providers? Instead, time and again, I was treated with nonchalance, indifference, or more rhetoric about how, *this is normal/just part of being a woman.*

Endometriosis.org (April, 2011) states "There is a significant diagnostic delay of endometriosis [of up to 12 years] because symptoms of the disease are not easily recognized in primary care – or even by women themselves." [19]

Unfortunately, there is no simple, easily recognizable test for Endometriosis. Testing for Endo is typically not a part of a woman's regular wellness care routine (e.g. pap-smear, breast exams, STD's, etc.) As noted by Endometriosis.org (2011), "At present the only reliable way to definitively diagnose endometriosis is by performing a laparoscopy and to take a biopsy of the tissue. This is what is known as 'the gold standard.'" [20]

The fact that there is not one all-encompassing, conclusive test for diagnosing Endometriosis is yet another frustrating piece of this astonishingly complicated puzzle. One might think, with all of the advances in modern medicine and science relative to women's health over the decades, that routine exams and tests to detect Endometriosis would be as commonplace as screenings for cancer. Sadly, for as far as we have come, we still have a long way to go. Right now, laparoscopy remains the foremost comprehensive method for diagnosis.

The Endometriosis Association (2007) states that,

> Diagnosis of Endo is generally considered uncertain until proven by laparoscopy – a surgical procedure done under anesthesia, where the patient's abdomen is distended with carbon dioxide gas to make the organs easier to see, and a laparoscope (a tube with a light in it) is inserted into a tiny incision in the abdomen. By moving the laparoscope around the abdomen, the surgeon can check the condition of the abdominal organs and, if careful and thorough, see the growths. A laparoscopy also indicates the locations, extent, and size of the growths and may help the doctor and patient make better –informed long-range decisions about treatment… [Although] a doctor can sometimes feel implants during a pelvic examination, and symptoms will often indicate Endo, it is not a good practice to treat this disease without confirmation of the diagnosis.' This is why laparoscopy is the best course of action for obtaining a proper diagnosis for endometriosis. [21]

While the proper procedure is crucial in obtaining a correct diagnosis, the proper medical professional is also critically imperative! Having the procedure performed by someone who is not specifically trained in the diagnosis or treatment of endometriosis can further exacerbate an already cryptic condition. It may also prevent you from receiving accurate information regarding your treatment and other options.

Endometriosis.org appears to agree that partnering with a trained Endo specialist is best, as they note:

> If the surgeon is not a specialist in endometriosis she/he may not recognize the disease, which can result in a "negative" result (e.g. you may be told that you have not got endometriosis, even if you do, because the surgeon was unable to visually recognize the disease, and[if] no biopsy was taken). [22]

Often times, the well-meaning medical professionals that women seek out to help them understand and make sense of the chaos happening inside their bodies, may simply lack the in-depth knowledge and education regarding Endometriosis that is necessary to give a fully informed, thorough and accurate diagnosis, and subsequent plan of treatment. Therefore, if you suspect you have endometriosis, I strongly encourage you to specifically seek out a medical professional who is not only an Endometriosis Specialist, but one who also has considerable expertise in reproductive and/or pelvic disorders. You should also do as much research and investigating of those topics as you can for yourself.

Treatments

One of the scariest revelations that I gleaned regarding my Endometriosis experience, one that I was not made aware of until after my surgery, is that THERE IS NO CURE FOR ENDOMETRIOSIS! In trying to help myself mentally decipher the turmoil that my body was experiencing, I envisioned *Endo* as being a 'glob' of 'something' inside my body that did not belong. In my ignorance, I thought that my surgery would basically consist of the doctors going in, removing the 'glob', and that following a few weeks of recovery time, I would be *'all good'!* If only things were that simple!

In my awareness advocacy efforts, I will sometimes come across women who may say, *"yeah, I had that"* or *" I remember when I used to have that."* Ladies, here me now and hear me well: while certain methods of treatment may cause an extended period of remission of symptoms, sometimes even for years, THERE IS NO

CURE FOR ENDOMETRIOSIS! There are, however, a variety of treatment options that can help you manage and alleviate symptoms, while greatly improving your quality of life. [23]

While treatment options are numerous, and vary greatly from woman to woman, they typically fall into one of four overall categories: pain management, hormonal therapy (used to shrink or slow endometrial growths), surgery, and complementary (alternative) treatment options.

Pain Management

With frequency, duration, and the severity of Endo-related pain varying so drastically from woman to woman, it would stand to reason that the type of drugs used for pain management would vary widely as well. Again, knowing that the amount and severity of pain doesn't always correlate to the staging and amount of Endo a woman has, there are some women with both minimal and advanced cases of Endo who can easily manage their pain symptoms with common over the counter or prescription medicines. The most commonly used medicines, are known as NSAID's (non-steroidal anti-inflammatory drugs), or what you may typically see sold as Ibuprofen (e.g. *Advil, Motrin,*), naproxen sodium (e.g. *Aleve, Naproxen*), and Mefenamic Acid (*Ponstan*). [24]

However, for many of us, the over-the-counter pain meds do absolutely nothing in the way of bringing us any level of significant relief. In fact, many Endo women experience levels of pain so excruciating that we are put on meds that fall into the category of opiates/narcotics. Furthermore, taking these types of medicines tend to put us into precarious situations for several reasons. For one, while these higher potency meds do tend to bring increased pain relief, they also pose a higher risk of negative side effects, along with an increased risk of developing chemical dependency. Another problem we face is that because many of these drugs are abused and sold illegally, it is often difficult for medical providers to believe the validity regarding the extent of our pain, and are often hesitant to fill prescriptions, especially if we tend to go through the prescription "too quickly."

Dilaudid, fentanyl, tramadol, Elavil, Neurontin, Norco, Ibuprofen 800 mg, Mefemamic Acid, are just a few of the medicines that I've had to endure over the years. In addition to these, other opiates/narcotics that are prescribed for Endo related pain include:

- Codeine

- Acetaminophen with Codeine (a.k.a. Tylenol 3)

- Morphine

- Methadone (a synthetic opiate)

- Hydrocodone (a.k.a. Vicodin, a.k.a. Lortab, a.k.a. Norco, a.k.a. Vicoprofen)

- Oxycodone (a.k.a. OxyContin, a.k.a. Percodan, a.k.a. Percoset). [25]

Some of the debilitating side effects associated with taking these meds, that are often minimized [when being prescribed], include: heavy fatigue, itchiness, suppressed breathing (feeling of suffocation), dizziness, irritability, anxiety, intense hunger or complete lack of hunger, headache, teeth grinding, hallucinations, depression, nausea, constipation. [26]

Some Endo sisters have also reported feeling: groggy, nauseated, and high. In addition, many have experienced symptoms of: vomiting, migrane headaches, and insomnia.

Often, it really is a *Catch-22* situation. It's like trading one set of f*cked up symptoms for a different set of even more f*cked up symptoms: having to choose between the lesser of two atrociously cruel evils. For example, either being in pain or dealing with the awful side-effects from the meds.

The Endometriosis Association summarizes the other main categories as follows:

HORMONAL THERAPY: Hormonal treatment aims to stop ovulation for as long as possible and may include: oral contraceptives, progesterone drugs, a testosterone derivative (danazol), and GnRH agonists (gonadotropin releasing hormone drugs[e.g. Luporn®]). [27]

Use of the drug Lupron® as a hormonal treatment for Endometriosis symptoms is often a hotly debated topic amongst Endo Sisters. In conversations with many women over the years, I've found that Lupron® is generally one of the first hormone based treatments prescribed to women as a treatment for Endometriosis. When it was offered to me, as a first course of treatment, what I didn't know was that it was originally developed to treat advanced prostate cancer in men. [23] In fact, had I known then what I know now about Lupron®, I would have never allowed it to be put into my body. While for many women it is an incredibly beneficial treatment that yields long lasting relief, my experience was quite the opposite.

While it was vaguely mentioned that I may experience some "slight, menopausal-type" symptoms, there was nothing slight about the reality of what I woefully endured during my six months of injections.

Terms such as hot flashes and dry mouth, were casually bantered about, but absolutely nothing was discussed about the potential for:

…tiredness, sweating, clamminess, breast tenderness, pain, change in breast size, vaginal discharge, dryness, itching, spotting (light vaginal bleeding), menstruation (periods), decrease in sexual ability/desire, swelling of the hands, feet, ankles, lower legs, pain, burning, tingling in the hands or feet, pain, burning, bruising, hardening at place where injection was given, change in weight, muscle or joint pain, flu-like symptoms, acne, depression, inability to control emotions, frequent mood changes, nervousness, general feeling of discomfort or uneasiness, difficulty with memory, itching, rash, or hives, difficulty breathing or swallowing, pain in the arms, back, chest, neck, or jaw, slow or difficult speech, dizziness or fainting, weakness, numbness, inability to move an arm or leg, bone pain, painful frequent or difficult urination, blood in urine, extreme thirst, weakness, dry mouth, nausea, vomiting, decreased consciousness, sudden headache, blurred vision, vision changes, difficulty moving eyes, drooping eyelids, and or confusion. [28]

Much to both my surprise and chagrin, I had to become intimately acquainted with many of these side-effects without any foreknowledge or insight. If I could do it over, I would have been more persistent in my refusal to consent to any form of treatment, until after I had completed a more in-depth and diligent self-study.

Please Note: This is not an attack against the use of *Lupron®*. I am speaking from my own personal experience. Every woman will respond to the treatment differently based on dosage and duration. Many woman have reported very positive results with the use of *Lupron®* as a way to manage their Endo symptoms. In contrast, I was simply was not one of them. In *Fighting Fiercely* for your own care, I lovingly urge you to get as much information as you can, so that you can make a fully informed decision before committing to any one form or any combination of treatment(s).

> **SURGERY:** Conservative surgery seeks to remove or destroy the growths, relieve pain, and may allow pregnancy to occur in some cases. Conservative surgery can involve laparoscopy (outpatient surgery in which the surgeon can view the inside of the abdomen through a tiny lighted tube that is inserted through one or more tiny abdominal incisions. Also referred to as "belly-button" surgery) or laparotomy (more extensive procedure, full incision, longer recovery period). Hormonal therapy may be prescribed along with conservative surgery. Radical surgery, which may be necessary in severe cases, involves: hysterectomy, removal of all growths, and removal of ovaries. [29]

> **ALTERNATIVE TREATMENTS:** Complementary treatment options may include: traditional Chinese medicine, nutritional approaches, homeopathy, allergy management, and immune therapy. [30]

No one treatment plan works for all women. Most women, myself included, often use a combination of treatments in order to find viable options for relief. I have, during the course of my own journey, utilized all of these treatment options at one time or another. Having multiple options at my disposal made the task of choosing a course of action a lot less daunting. There was a particular peace of mind in knowing that as my symptoms changed, so could my options for treatment.

CHAPTER 3
THE DESTRUCTION...
AND THE AFTER MATH

"Things jus' ain't the same." ~Dr. Dre.

In the weeks leading up to my surgery, I was faced with an onslaught of mental, physical, and emotional adjustments that needed to be made, as my mother would say, *"quick, fast, and in a hurry!"* Having just moved only a few months prior, I was still pretty much living out of boxes, and had to prepare my place with everything that I would need for my aftercare. As I lived alone, and would be on bed rest for several weeks afterward, I needed to organize my sleeping space for maximum comfort and easy access to the things that I would need. I would have to stock up on food (that would be easy to prepare), first aid, and many personal hygiene items that I would need for both pre-and-post surgery prep.

Having just secured a wellness contract with a huge client, I still had to get my staff hired and trained, before taking my medical leave. In addition, I needed to continue preparing my body for surgery by keeping up with all of the hormones, pain killers, and vitamins that I had to take several times a day while battling the side effects. Most days I felt like a character in a Spike Lee movie-you know in the scenes where they are supposed to be walking down the street, but they actually look as if they're floating in midair-yeah, that was me. In fact, trying to manage the emotional side effects was as much a challenge as trying to manage my pain.

March 8th, 2008

Today is a ho-hum kinda day....I know ho-hum is generic and corny, but I can't really think of another way to describe it. There is still one week and three days until my surgery and I'm really starting to get annoyed with the whole thing. The past couple days, my vagina has been dry and irritated as hell, but I suppose that can happen when you've been wearing pads/panty-liners and bleeding for 32 days!! FINALLY, the spotting has tapered off some, so I said f*ck it and went commando last night and all of today! Hell, my kitty kat needed a breather! Like Clay Davis [from The Wire] would say – "SHEEEEEEEEEEIIIIIIIT"- you know I can't stand wearing no panties!!! Hell with all that's going on – with feeling so captive to this whole freakin process – I ain't felt so free in weeks! Sh*t, my arms and wrists are STILL bruised from needles stuck in my arms four weeks ago! Thank GOD I never tried to take up the life of a dope fiend – with these lil tiny rollin' viens – I never woulda been any good at it! It'll probably be well into summer before I get my normal color back! On top of that, this stint is starting to aggra-vate the hell outta me – got me reverting back to when it was first put in – the frequent urge to pee – most time with little or no fluid or worse a trickle here or a few drops there. And my back!!!! In a constant state of tremendous soreness due to the constant spasms every time I pass fluid. My glutes and piriformis are so tight! To make matters worse, to complicate my vaginal irritation - I AM HORNY AS HELL! Which in essence, is a good thing, and I suppose I shouldn't be complaining about it - 'cuz one of the side effects of all these meds is supposed loss of sex drive – so I guess I should be happy for that? Add to that, the swelling and fullness and tenderness of my breasts (which btw they also said they could possibly decrease [in size] – but thank God they did not)…..if I had a husband here to quench that fire, but alas, I don't so…..to make matters worse than the extent of my physical issues – emotional-ly…..I'm still just…..

Tuesday, March 18th

Tomorrow is my surgery – its finally here. And honestly, I don't really feel any particular thing about it one way or the other. I'm glad I'm on the road to this-is-almost-over-ness! People keep askin' "how you feel?', are u scared?, and are you nervous?" To be hon-est, I really don't feel anything, I'm really just kinda matter-of -fact about it. I'm really just kinda like let's go in and get it over with and get on with the business of getting on with it! I've reached out to all the people who matter and they've reached out to me. We've all touched, prayed, agreed, lifted up, pleaded the Blood, strapped on our Spiritual armor, now we're armed and ready to go! So, let's go get this thing over with! Dad is here at the house with me, and *mom is meeting us at the hospital – we gotta be there at 6am, the surgery is scheduled for 7:30 am. I suppose I should get some sleep, it's gonna be a long day tomorrow...Prayerfully, this will all be over soon and I will be back on the road to fabulosity-ness!*

After thoroughly discussing the extent of the damage the disease had caused in my body, along with future options and plans for fertility and pregnancy, my medical team and I opted for excision surgery. We decided to use the *Da Vinci* ® robotic excision method in order to remove my chocolate cyst (tumor), as well as, other endometrial implants, lesions, and adhesions from the affected areas. Because I still planned to have children, I did not want any surgical options that would include destroying my uterine lining (ablation) or the removal of my uterus and/or ovaries (hysterectomy). Unfortunately, because the disease had so significantly infested the left side of my reproductive system, I had no choice but to have my left ovary and fallopian tube removed. However, by retaining my right ovary and tube, I was still able to preserve my chances for childbearing.

I felt most comfortable in choosing the *Da Vinci* ® method, because, after researching several surgical options I found that with this method, as outlined on davincisurgery.com,

> Surgeons operate through a few small incisions instead of a large open incision – similar to traditional laparoscopy. The *Da Vinci* System features a magnified 3D high-definition vision system and special wristed instruments that bend and rotate far greater than the human wrist. As a result, *Da Vinci* enables your surgeon to operate with enhanced vision, precision, dexterity and control... *Da Vinci's* 3D HD vision system allows surgeons to see key anatomy with depth and clarity– critical to removing deep endometrial tissue implants. State-of-the-art *Da Vinci* uses the latest in surgical and robotics technologies and is beneficial for performing complex surgery. Your surgeon is 100% in control of the *Da Vinci* System, which translates his or her hand movements into smaller, more precise movements of tiny instruments inside your body. [31]

I had endured so many smaller surgeries and procedures

leading up to the excision, one of my foremost concerns was the overlapping recovery that would result from this more extensive surgery. After researching other surgical methods, I became most comfortable with the *Da Vinci* ® method as based on the particular benefits that are listed on davincisurgery.com, the more promising of which include:

- **Low blood loss**

- **Low conversion rate to open surgery**

- **Low rate of complications**

- **Short hospital stay**

- **Small incisions for minimal scarring.** [32]

Please Note: I just want to take a moment to say that my decision to use this particular method for my treatment is not an endorsement for *Da Vinci,* nor an indictment against any other method for treatment. Based on the specifics of my particular diagnosis, along with my personal goals for quality of life, career, and family, this was the best option for me. Before making any decision regarding surgery or any other treatment option, I would strongly urge you to educate and equip yourself with as much information from as many reliable sources as you can, on as many options as you can. Research, compare-and-contrast the benefits, as well as the risks, and the long-term outcomes as it relates to your own future goals for quality of life, career, and family. Investigate your surgeons by researching their expertise with different methods and patient satisfaction with their practices.

Whatever method for surgery or treatment you choose, my sincerest hope for you is that your decision is one that is wholly, thoroughly, and completely comfortable, reasonable, and acceptable for you. It should be one that allows you to be educated, enlightened, and empowered as a proactive participant in your decision.

I'm not quite sure if it was denial, shock, the remnants of anesthesia still coursing through my veins, or just the normal course of post-surgical recovery; but in the days and weeks immediately following my surgery, I found myself mentally, physically and emotionally blank. With the exception of my parents, I basically cut myself off from the world, and began to retreat inside myself. While I know that my friends and family were simply concerned about me and wanted to make sure I was progressing well in my recovery, the truth is, I didn't want to be bothered. I didn't want any visitors. I didn't want any well-wishers. I didn't want any help. All I wanted to do is sleep, hoping on some subconscious level that when I finally awoke, all of this would have been nothing more than some awful, terrible, horrible dream. And alas, though I did sleep, often for several days at a time, every sharp, stabbing, gnawing pain that would jar me awake served as an all too real reminder that this was in fact, no dream at all! My biggest reality check came the first time I caught a glimpse of my freshly stitched wounds in the mirror.

March 2009

Truth be told, I never wanted to be skinny! More than that, I never wanted to be one of those girls with the six pack abs or a washboard stomach! I actually loved my lil' tummy pooch! To me, there was always something inherently soft and feminine, sexy and nurturing, delicate and "just so" about my slightly protruding, fluffy lil soft spot. It was the kind that was made for caressing, fondling, cuddling and holding. It was my center, my core, my gut-check, my radar; it was the house that guarded my solar plexus; my anchor, my Spirit. It was that safe and sacred space that would hold and protect my children as they were shaped, knit, and formed inside my womb. It was always his favorite pillow. That peaceful, private place where Mista could always rest his head. If you looked ever so closely, you could still see the faint outline of my birthmark, floating just above my belly button. But now, standing here reflecting, I realized I was just a shadow of my former self – cut, scarred, discolored, ripped open and stitched back together – jagged pieces of string yanked and pulled across my once upon-a-time smooth and creamy skin. All I felt now was… FAT… horrid, and empty… hollow, busted, bloated, bruised, and…B-R-O-K-E-N!

I don't remember how long I stood there looking in that mirror. My wounds and I were weeping together. I don't remember cleaning or changing the dressing. I definitely don't remember how or when I crawled back into bed. What I do remember, is that at some point, when the pools of tears clouded my vision (so much that I could no longer see), I stopped even trying to. I simply closed my eyes…and I slept.

April 19th, 2008

One month ago today, my life changed – well, not that my life hadn't been changing – I mean, it actually started closer to three months ago, at the end of December – when I thought I had the stupid flu! But, a month ago, four weeks ago this past Wednesday, another episode of change occurred in my life. I had gone in to have the surgery for my endometriosis. I thought it was simple enough. They went in, removed my diseased, scarred fallopian tube and ovary from my left side, along with all the cysts. They removed another smaller cyst from my right fallopian tube, drained the fluid out, and left all else intact. And at first, I thought that was all there was to it. [I thought] I'd be down for a couple weeks and before long, I'd be back to business. Simple enough, right ? However, during my first post–op visit I was told that: the disease was more wide-spread than first thought, more intertwined and intermixed with pelvic tissues, structures, and nerves which would have been much more dangerous for them to try to cut around or remove it. So alas, I still have deposits of it left in me. As a result, I have another three more months of the horrible Luporn therapy, followed by on-going birth control therapy. The hope is that any residual disease will 'dissolve' and my estrogen levels will stay low enough, so as not to have a reoccurrence of the cysts / growths. (Hopefully, they say. I honestly don't think they have any real f*ckin' clue as to whether or not this will actually work. But, we shall see).

Even after the surgery, I still had to keep that stupid stint in my kidneys which became an absolutely unbearable pain after a while. When I got it out two weeks later, it was such a relief! Physically and emotionally, I still felt anesthetized – even suffering from a brief moment of pseudo wellness – when I was so doped up and feeling 'no pain', I actually went to the store and carried groceries home…and stretched [my body into weird positions] trying to *polish my toenails with sexy red polish. I was fine until reality set in [and the meds wore off] and my pelvis started to feel like it was on fire! That day was insanely bad for me! When the pain resurfaced, I panicked! It felt like I was being ravaged all over again from the inside out! I felt afflicted with a consuming wave of fear and I just burst out crying uncontrollably. I just kept hearing in my head over-and -over again, "stupid b*tch! You f*cked up!" I just kept hearing over-and-over again that I would never be able to have children! And as hard as I tried to push it down or pray it away, those thoughts just kept consuming me and I couldn't stop crying! I didn't know what else to do…after that, I parked myself on my sofa sleeper and did not move for a week!*

Moving into week three[post-op], I'm slowly starting to back off the narcotics and ease off the IB 800's. I'm starting to take my iron pills and vitamins every day and my 'add-back' medicine to help ward off some of the hot flashes – sometimes it works, sometimes it doesn't…I think on some level I've been drowning my fears and insecurities in food – knowingly eating all kinds of unhealthy sh*t and being seriously hungry at odd times of the night – it could be the insomnia I'm often stricken with. But I'm hoping it'll wane once I'm back on my regular schedule… it's still hard sometimes sleeping alone while I deal with this, and I'm thinking of joining a support group, because my emotions do drift sometimes…

As the days continued to pass, I found myself battling with a myriad of emotions and thoughts that often were conflicting and condescending. I half-heartedly went through the motions during: follow-up doctor's appointments, modified bathing, walking, and sleeping rituals. Although I was present physically, the gravity of what I had gone through still hadn't actually resonated with me emotionally. It still hadn't sank in, so, mentally and emotionally, I checked out. There was also the realization that the surgery didn't "fix" everything. In fact, pieces of this disease were still left lurking inside me, waiting to attack and snatch what life was left out of me at any moment! The heaviness made me feel as if all the drugs, meds, injections, and side effects were pointless! Why suffer through this personal hell, if there was still a chance that after: all the pain, soreness, poking, prodding, cutting, scraping, stitching, insomnia, night sweats, hair loss, crying, depression, confusion, and isolation that I could end up repeating this whole process. If, I was only going to end up in another hospital bed, on another surgery table, or go through all of this again…then what the was the point of having done it at all?

The weight that I carried in my mind and heart eventually began to show up on my body. I was confined to bed rest, with limited mobility, and physically incapacitated to the point of not being able to share more than a phone call or a text message with friends or family (not wanting to do much more than that honestly). As the days passed I was trapped in the house, by myself, feeling isolated, lost, and very much alone. I felt helpless to control the side effects and did not understand how these drugs that were supposed to be helping me were seemingly doing more harm than good.

Incapable of managing so many of the things going on in my life, one of the few things I could control, even if in a subconscious sense, was food! Before Endometriosis wrought havoc on my life, I was only nine pounds away from my goal weight. By the time I was six months post-op, I had picked up an additional 30 pounds! Being so physically limited in the beginning, I was not able to stand for long periods of time, so cooking wasn't a top priority. At first it was more for convenience, but over time, all the frozen foods and "quick-fix" meals (e.g. breads, pizza, pasta, subs, Chinese, Mexican, Italian take-out) became more of a comfort in my dark, lonely, hours of insomnia. Hell, what did it matter anymore? My life was sh*t! I felt like I didn't have anybody in my life before this and I certainly wouldn't find anybody now. Who was going to want an over 30, overweight, half barren chick with scarred body parts, who was also suffering, from chemically induced menopause, adult acne, and missing clumps of her hair? Not a single damned soul would, I thought. So f*ck it! If a pan of brownies and a quart of vanilla bean ice cream, a large everything pizza, a pan of fries, and a salad to reconcile it all was going to comfort me in my time of need, then so be it!

Several more weeks schlepped on with more of the same, but eventually, things slowly began to get better. Much like the pleasant change in seasons from colder to warmer months, so went the changes in my physical and emotional disposition. With each passing day, the scars gradually began to heal, the bruises began to dissipate, the fatigue faded away, and my energy crept back. Soon, I would be returning to my exciting, albeit physically demanding career. Therefore, I began to exercise in preparation to build up my stamina. Nothing crazy or too intense, just a slow walk in the park for about 15 minutes, one or two days a week. Then I progressed to strolling on the lakefront for about 30 minutes, nearly every day. I savored feeling the warmth of the sun, the breeze on my skin, the fresh air in my nostrils, and watching the ebb and flow of calming waves on the beach. Walking on the lakeshore, did more to brighten my spirits than even I could have imagined. Though still pretty thin, my hair had finally stopped falling out, and thanks to the miracle working hands, and razor sharp scissors of the world's greatest hairdresser (Hey, Sunito), I was even starting to feel a faint stirring of that soft, dare I say sexy femininity that I thought would forever be lost.

May 13, 2008

...This past Saturday I finally got my hair done after six months of drama and trauma! It felt and looked so good by the time I left, I said Hell, just call me New-New [the lead female character from the movie ATL], cuz I feel like a New New woman!

Nearly two months out of surgery, it spontaneously occurred to me, *"Damn, I might finally get through this after all."*

June 23rd 2008

...In other news, I finally got my last hormone injection! Woooo Hooo! Thank G-O-D! Now, we move into phase II of this post-operative out-patient therapy! When I had my visit on the 16th, we discussed that, overall, it seemed as if I'd tolerated the Lupron fairly well (hot flashes, migraines, hair loss, and weight gain aside-insert sarcasm here); The suppression of the Endo symptoms seemed to be being handled pretty well. So, at this point I can now switch to continual birth control therapy which will still control my symptoms without the [hot] flashes, migraines, etc. She told me to get over the counter prenatal vitamins for the hair loss and to boost my vitamin B... I start all that on July 13th and then after a month, I check in with her to see how they are working. All things con-

sidered, I think I'll be okay. I did have a slight scare this Friday and Saturday with an increase in pain. I think I pushed myself a little too hard with the working out...But I have been continually faithful to my workouts 4-5 times a week, despite the fact that the numbers on the scale keep going up! I keep gaining weight! I'm hoping that this whole hormonal business is a contributing factor and once that subsides, my work will start to show in the numbers. Plus, I'm gonna start adding some strength training to the game to see if that helps.....we shall see!

CHAPTER 4
RE-SET... REBOUND

"It a'int ovah" ~Guy.

After moving into *Phase II* of my treatment, I believed I was beginning to regain my sense of "pre- Endo" normalcy. I had returned to work with a refreshed sense of excitement and vigor. Our corporate client was now interested in expanding our ground-breaking wellness program. I had become more consistent with my workouts, and had even begun to ease back into a social life with some of my closest friends. Of course, I would have some bad days, where my motivation would surpass my physical ability, and I'd extend myself a bit too aggressively, and find myself needing a day or two to recover. Not being on the hormones anymore was a huge relief, as I personally felt, despite what doctors said, that they were not the biggest factor in bringing me any relief. They sure as hell were not worth the tradeoff of side effects. Two months without them, I had a renewed sense of clarity, (no more brain fog or forgetfulness) and I felt my productivity increasing daily. Admittedly, whenever I would have a pain spike, or light spotting, or any type of increased physical discomfort, I would panic, and my mind would drift back to the worst memories from months earlier. Sometimes the scare would last a few hours; sometimes a few days. Each time, I would try to remind myself that I had nothing to worry about, this was all a part of the healing process, that things were going well, and that I was going to be fine. And I was, until...

August 15th, 2008

Today I was diagnosed with clinical depression. I'm so overwhelmed right now- my head hurts. I can't even process this right now. C-L-I-N-I-C-A-L D-E-P-R-E-S-S-I-O-N – WTF!? I can't even write about it anymore.

August 19th, 2008

So, I'm still trying wrap my mind around this "clinical depression" deal. After having some time to take it all in, I can see where it makes sense. I've had so much going on...everything just col-

lapsed on top of itself and I feel like I'm drowning! I don't even know what happened; one minute I was [in the doctor's office] discussing my recovery, the next minute I was on the floor, this uncontrollable weeping, and sobbing mess! I'm too embarrassed to even think about the things that I admitted to the social worker. I think I'd shoot myself if I wrote them down to be read out loud. I couldn't bear to have that information roaming around in the universe, staring back at me, and one day possibly being read by someone else. Hell, I can't even admit that I've actually admitted to half the sh*t I admitted to – if that even makes and sense? But, after it was over, the "evaluation" I mean, she said I was "textbook" and that I should see someone right away.

Wednesday, August 20, 2008

Today is not such a good day. But I'm at work, so I'm putting up a hard front. I don't think those [depression] meds are helping much. I'm up now more in the middle of the night than I was before! The racing thoughts have slowed down some but – I still don't feel like my old self! I'm still trying to find a stupid "therapist'" and if I knew it was this hard…I'm starting to wonder if this is even what I really need? Is this even going to help me? So far, I haven't noticed any stellar difference. Saturday – nothing, Sunday – a little nauseous, Monday – pretty down, I sent Esther in to work for me. That was a bad day! I cried all over the place. Yesterday, I wanted to crawl in bed and stay there all day, but I couldn't. I had a meeting [with our client] so I feigned my way through that as best I could. Came home, I managed to get through dinner and get to bed, but I'll be damned if I wasn't up tossing and turning in a matter of hours …

August 21st 2008

Today, I wanted to crawl under the covers and just stay there all day doing nothing – but then I knew if I did I would only feel guilty and torture myself all day…so I said f*ck it – I dragged myself up, and forced myself to make it to my one saving grace- my job! Now, most people feel the exact opposite about their place of employment, but me, I have to say I love what I do! It's the one place where I can come and for a few hours, push all of my crap to the side and focus on someone else and actually feel good about helping others, which in turn makes me feel good about myself. It's the journey to get to work that's the kicker! It is such a struggle to actually get out the door, to actually get motivated to MOVE! Today I actually sat around until 11:30 before I even tried to take a shower, let alone do anything else...I've only told five people about the diagnosis. I kinda wish I hadn't told Connie, but she's my coordinator [at the corporate site], and this is affecting my work, so I had to tell her. I don't think anyone else [at the site] would understand. Before I realized what was actually wrong with me – I remember telling my friends, and talking to people saying, "I'm not happy with this or I'm frustrated with this or that, I'm sad, I'm depressed." In response, everybody said I was over-reacting or that it wasn't that bad...I finally got a call back from one of the counseling centers (YEAH) I got an appointment for Monday, the 25th at 10am – FINALLY! Maybe now I can uproot some of these disparaging feelings from my life....we shall see.

August 24, 2008

Today I'm very sad and I don't even really know why. My birthday is exactly one week from today and I should be really psyched about it, but I'm not. One of my closest, best friends is getting married in a little more than two weeks and I get to go visit California for the first time, and I' not even excited about that either! I have been feeling like a freaking zombie all day! I didn't go to church and I felt nauseated most of the day. I've been having pain on my right side again. Tomorrow is my first day in therapy and I should be excited about that- about getting help, about getting out of this funk! I just feel so blah! I'm not really feeling motivated to do more or do anything in particular. I'm sick of this medication. I don't feel like it's doing anything. I just want to go back to feeling like myself. To be normal! Shoot, I don't even feel like writing anymore!

Wednesday. August 27th, 2008

Today feels like a pretty decent day so far...I guess I'm doing okay. I didn't have much of a struggle getting out of the house as I had been and I slept pretty soundly last night for a change. On Monday (the 25th) I had my first therapy session. It was okay I guess. My therapist Maureen, my God, I can't even believe I said *that, my T-H-E-R-A-P-I-S-T seems like a pretty nice lady and she was relatively easy to talk to. Of course, I ran my mouth the whole time, but hell, that's what I was supposed to do...*

I can't really say when or at what point the disconnect happened. For a time, I really did think I was okay. Looking back, I was clearly repressing my feelings about the experience thus far, and catapulting all my energies into "getting back to my old self." In hindsight, I truly believed that if I didn't think about it, if I didn't focus on it, if I ignored the little pings and twangs of pain that would constantly nag and prick me, if I threw myself with restless vigor into all my "pre-Endo" activities...then somehow, the past eight months really wouldn't be real, everything that happened to me really wouldn't have happened. Clearly, I wasn't trying to deal with it! But at some point, all the stifling, and ignoring, and pushing down became futile. Sooner rather than later, I was going to have to deal with the festering emotional and mental wounds that were getting worse, even as my physical wounds continued to heal. And sooner came that day in my doctor's office, when my emotions, and my tears all came spilling out; at the same time, all over the exam room floor...there was no more running, no more hiding, no more pretending. My Endometriosis was REAL, my surgery and all of its after effects were REAL, and it was affecting my life in very real ways. It was about time I started equipping myself with some very REAL tools to accept it and deal with it.

Working with the therapist over the next few weeks proved to be incredibly powerful for me in regaining clarity, focus, and control in not only fully accepting the changes that I'd gone through, but also in addressing the fear that had completely paralyzed me. First, in getting over the fear of the *"Black People don't do therapy"* stigma, I realized that it was also the fear of how much I didn't know about Endometriosis, even after all I'd been through up to this point, that was holding me hostage to my increasingly detrimental depression. Working with the therapist to confront those fears also empowered me to become accountable for my own awareness. I needed to learn as much as I could about this disease, how it had affected me, and what I could do to take back my life! Being the textbook Virgo that I am, I became a research renegade, scouring the internet for as much information as I could find about Endo.

Not just about the pathology of the disease, but about the mental, physical, and emotional impact that it has on one's life. I began to seek out other women's stories and experiences. The research and information I found, helped me learn more than what the doctors had given me. This information wasn't just recited from some text-book or case study, this information rang true to *my* specific experience and it did wonders in helping to ease the anxiety, lessen the fears, and curb the depression. As time went on, I started to get better. Not just on the surface, but deep down inside.

Wednesday, September 17ᵗʰ, 2008

Today was a really good day! I'm not sure why, but I actually felt good today. Besides my normal sluggishness in getting up so early, but other than that, I felt more like my normal self today than I have in a long time – longer than I can remember! It wasn't a chore to get out of the house – I was actually looking forward to going to work. I actually saw the sunshine and enjoyed the warmth for the first time in a long time. I actually felt like myself. I felt normal, I felt…. H-A-P-P-Y! Today was a good day!

September 27ᵗʰ, 2008 Saturday

Today, I went outside, I know that sounds like a small, trivial nothing, but for me, considering where I've been, it's a milestone, because I am not outside going to work, or running errands or doing something out of necessity, but I'm out – at the beach, in front of the water - in my most favorite place with my feet in the sand and the wind in my hair and the sun at my back and the breeze on my face. And for once I feel….somewhat free. GOD – I hadn't been outside in so long. I can't believe I let the whole summer pass and I didn't spend more time here…

For the next two months, things were good. Not perfect, but good. I had finally managed to positively assert my new definition of "normal" into my life. This meant: incorporating my new rituals of daily meds, symptom journaling, and easing back into social and physical activities. I continued with therapy. I also continued to educate, enlighten, and empower myself in every way that I could about every facet of endometriosis and its effects.

Then, in what I would come to know as a hallmark characteristic of this unpredictable disease, just as I was starting to get comfortable, thinking that I'd finally had a secure grasp on the nature of this *beast*...

November 8th, 2008

BAD NEWS – I've been spotting now for almost two doggone weeks! I panicked when it first started, but the doctors assured me that this was "normal" and that sometimes when you use the pill continuously you may have "breakthrough bleeding", which I suppose wouldn't be so bad if I didn't have this excruciating pain to go along with it! I'm not even bleeding heavily, but with these cramps, you'd think I was bleeding a river! I'm just ready for it to STOP already! I go in next Friday to get checked out, so we'll see what happens. I hope I'm not having a set back! I don't think I could take it, especially when things are going so well and finally starting to turn around for me. I don't think I could take any devastation of that magnitude. Not now, hell, not ever after going through what I went through this past year...

November 25th, 2008

...I'm also rethinking about joining that support group for endometriosis. I've been spotting and cramping for about the past three weeks and when I went to the Obgyn this past Friday, she said she felt a small mass: a nodule of some sort behind my cervix. She's scheduled me for another ultrasound just to make sure there's nothing wrong. I'm trying not to go into panic mode about it...guess we'll just have to wait and see what happens...

I was trying, Lord knows I was trying…. to keep in mind all the tools I'd gained in therapy to combat the impending cloud of fear that had begun looming overhead and in my gut. I tried to tell myself that it had only been nine months since my surgery and with an experience of that magnitude, it will take some time for the body to completely heal. And with all the continued "aftercare" I was going through, it would probably take much more time than I was allowing myself. I tried to convince myself to calm down, to not push myself, to be patient with myself…but somewhere, deep down inside of me, I couldn't escape what I knew. I couldn't ignore the fact that, despite their best efforts, the doctors weren't able to remove all of the disease. It was still there, prowling around my insides, lurking about near delicate nerves and connective structures, knowing it would be too dangerous to attempt to excise from those areas. The last thing doctors wanted to do was assume the perilous risk of causing me paralysis or even worse, causing me to bleed out. It was still there, just waiting to slither its way to what was left of my reproductive organs and strangle what life had remained there waiting to come forth. I knew… and all the coping skills in the world wouldn't make that go away. But I still tried…

Thursday, December 9th, 2008

So, the past few days of my life have been eventful to say the least! Last Tuesday (the 2nd) I went to have my ultrasound! I was nervous I admit, and I was not too happy when I left. Of course, the technicians themselves could not state anything directly to me about what they found, however, I did overhear them talking amongst each other. I kept hearing words float through the air like: 'cyst', 'fluid', 'old blood…' they asked me at least three times if I'd had a history of fibroids in my family, and that lead me to definitely believe that they saw SOMETHING; although what exactly, I'm not sure. I'm scheduled to find out more this Friday when I go for my follow up. 'Til then, I'm trying not to let my mind get away from me with all sorts of malicious thoughts. This hasn't been easy since I've been in pain since they started poking and digging around up there. I've stopped bleeding though, so that's good! But the pain got so bad last night, I had to take more Norco! It didn't shut it down quite like I expected so, I might have to take two, and go to bed early. I am concerned, but it's not at the high level of anxiety as before. This time, I knew what the heck was wrong with me! I've got more of a peace about things. This time, it's more of let's find out what's wrong, so we can get on about the business of correcting it…

Wednesday, December 17th, 2008

I got the results of my ultrasound back – and they did find, what they say is a "very small" fibroid tumor. They say it's not even as big as a golf ball, so at this point, it's nothing to worry about (although I'm not so sure about all that). They also found a small ovarian cyst on my right side; it is one of the "normal" fluid filled

45

ones that will either dissolve or pass through the body on its own. As for the pain...with Endo (they say) there can be "flare-ups", so I've just had to ramp up my regimen of meds until I can get the pain under control again. So, I'm happy. Not too thrilled about the meds, but I'm happy it was nothing too major or serious.

January 16th, 2009

In other news – Monday (January 12th) was my last session with the therapist WOOOOOO HOOOO! My bout with clinical depression is o-v-e-r! At least that's what the therapist says! For now at least. I still need to have a final evaluation with the psychiatrist to get released from the meds – until then, I have to keep pushing the Prozac....but at least I'm on my way.

As it turned out, Black people do *"do therapy."* The coping skills I gained in working with the therapist actually proved surprisingly useful in the days and weeks to come. For example, I was able to recognize these new developments clearly and calmly, without the cloud of fear looming overhead. I was able to work proactively, both on my own and with my medical and mental professionals to manage the situation as best as I could without it overtaking me and unraveling all the progress I had made. I was no longer willing to be held captive by this "thing", so I reached down deep, mustered up the remnants of all the strength I had left, and decided: I AM GOING TO GET THROUGH THIS!

CHAPTER 5
RELAPSE... RECOVER

"Here we go again..." ~Chuck D.

Get through it is exactly what I did. I was determined to regain my "pre-Endo" sense of normalcy. When I realized that would never be possible, as my life had forever been changed by it, I decided to redefine my sense of "post-Endo" normalcy instead. For example, rather than dread taking my medications, I mentally added them as just another practice in my daily routine. In fact, I added them right along with my journaling, prayers, and exercise routine. I was back to eating healthier and to working out more consistently. I was even taking kickboxing and African dance classes! I worked when I needed to work and rested when I needed to rest. I ended my nights early or started my days later when I needed to adapt. I kept my meds on me at all times. I had even figured out a system of being pre-emptive with my pain management meds, so, that I wouldn't "crash" on the days that I knew would be more physically strenuous. I was cautiously dedicated to my Endo journal, taking meticulous care to record any changes, patterns or anomalies in the manifestations of my symptoms.

My career could not have been better! We received yet a third expansion of our corporate wellness program, including: a two year extension on our contract and a compensation increase of $25,000! I had just hired my second employee and he could not have been a more perfect fit! I was back to hanging out and "kicking it" with my girls on a regular basis! Hell, I had even started dating someone! Life was finally good again! After nearly a year, my suppression regimen seemed to be holding up, and I was finally settling into my new definition of normal. While no longer in denial about my new Endo-infused reality, I also wasn't depressed or being held hostage by it either! Most of time, I could go all day with little-to-no pain. And when those days became weeks, and those weeks became a few consecutive months, I became so enthralled with living my life, I had almost forgot that I had it! Almost......

Sunday, December 13th, 2009

It is a wonder how much a person's life can change in just a matter of days! The next morning after my last entry (12/09/09, Wednesday) after a night of tumultuous bleeding and cramping and passing blood clots that looked like someone had dumped jars of grape jelly into my panties, I found myself in the ER at Northwestern Memorial Hospital with the same symptoms that showed up 18 months ago when I was first diagnosed with Endometriosis – after 4 hours of more testing and more diagnosis – they found yet another tumor/cyst/Endometrioma – along with more fluid buildup in my right and dare I say only present and working fallopian tube which means another damn surgery! As soon as possible is what they say! Unfortunately, I can't even get in a follow-up appointment to set the date for the surgery until 12/23/09. That's more than two weeks away! So, I'm stuck with the incessant bleeding and cramping and overall f*cked-up-ness for another two weeks before they decide what to do with me! I'm not panicked, I'm not freaked out, I'm just frustrated! And Pissed! It's taken me just this long to finally recapture some semblance of normalcy to my life! My diet, my exercise, my confidence, my self-esteem, all of it – I was finally starting to feel normal again – NOW, here we go again with this sh*t!

I could not believe it! I was absolutely floored! The entire foundation of everything I'd built over the past 18 months crumbled right before me in a matter of moments! All of the memories, all the pain, all the emotions, all the trauma, all of it poured over me like waves crashing with the force of a tsunami! My first thought was that I could not go through this again! Physically, mentally, emotionally, I couldn't…no way in hell-or-heaven for that matter would I be able to endure another 18 months of what I'd just recovered from. Now I was laying there, almost two years to the date of when I'd began to have my initial onset of symptoms. Now I was in that same emergency room, wearing that same paper thin gown, ass and cooch exposed again for a brand new sh*tload of strangers: to see, stick, poke, prod, examine, assess, suppose and hypothesize about me all over again. All I could think about were those stereotypical people we joke about who are always overacting at funerals; the ones who take one peek in the casket and start wailing and screaming and falling out. The ones always exclaiming: *"Aw Lawd Sweet Jeeeezus! Whyyyyyyy Lawd, whhhhhyyy Jeszus!!! Take ME Lawd!!! Just take me nah!"* Yeah, that was me, now.

??? 2009

People are always saying to me *"You're so strong, brave, and independent."* You think I do sh*t alone because I want to! No, it's because I have to!!! I'm about to have to go through all this surgery crap a-g-a-i-n - alone, and by myself!!! Do you know how much that sucks! But, I did it the last time, I guess I'll do it this time...

Thursday, December 24th, 2009

Well, it's Christmas Eve – again, Another year has passed and here I sit alone – again! Yesterday I got the most devastating news. I went to the follow up from my ER visit, and to put it bluntly, the doctors basically feel like it's not worth it to go through such a risky procedure with such a long recovery period and expose me to the formation of more adhesions and scar tissue for a 2cm endometriomial cyst; only to have me come back in another 18 months or so for yet another surgery. She feels like it's too big a risk and basically feels like we'll get into a cycle of doing this over-and-over again. Her solution: she doesn't think my symptoms will ever completely subside or I'll be pain free unless and until they go in and take everything out and by everything I mean all my reproductive parts(i.e. hysterectomy - they really seem to like pushing that shit) so that I'll not be able to have children. Well, I promptly dismissed that and asked what about my non-surgical options. *"Not Many"* she said. [what the hell???] As a doctor, she says that her team is basically stuck and they DON'T KNOW WHAT TO DO WITH ME! Before deciding to do anything she said she wants to wait another two weeks for another, more clear ultrasound to see what's really going on (but what the fuck does it matter if you don't know what to do with me?) Then, she said she wants to refer me to this [doctor] in Evanston, Illinois who is supposed to be a pelvic pain specialist. They said I may be able to get a second opinion or other options. In addition to that, she changed my meds AGAIN back to a 30mg birth control pill this time. So, now, I've got to *take: birth control pills, ibuprophen pills, Norco, and some new meds, (that's actually an anti-depressant), but is also used to treat chronic pain. I start tonight so we'll see what happens. So, I get to do this regimen for about a month or so, then I check back in- this whole wait and see approach sucks! Meanwhile I'm going to ask her if they can at least drain the fluid from my tube to see if that will at least help in alleviating the pain! In the meantime, we're stuck with more wait and see. What kind of bullshit is this!?*

WE-DON'T- KNOW- WHAT- TO- DO- WITH YOU.... WE-DON'T-KNOW- WHAT- TO- DO- WITH YOU.... Those words echoed in my head over and over again. Who in *seven hells* sanctioned this type of foolishness! How can you NOT know what else to do with me? YOU are the doctors! YOU are the professionals! YOU went to school for years and years. You spent all that money to put all those accolades and letters behind your name! How the hell can you NOT KNOW what else to do with me? What kind of half-wit, dumb asses were these people? Frustrated was an understatement! I was absolutely mortified! I was beginning to feel just like them, because hell, at this point I didn't know what to do with me either. There was one thing I did know, I was not about to let this new development drag me back down the dark hole of despair from which I had just spent the last 18 months freeing myself.

So, I took a breath, took a moment, and allowed myself to become still. I sat there, breathing and quiet, clearing my head of all the mental clutter and internal chatter. Once I commanded my emotions to settle down, I took a mental step back and re-evaluated the situation by looking only at the facts. First, this disease isn't going anywhere. Despite all best efforts thus far, it has resurfaced, and now poses another potential threat. Second, the current medical team that I am working with have exhausted all of their options in the realm of their expertise, (which I feel is clearly limited as it relates to Endometriosis). Third, there are more doctors with a wider, greater, more extensive scope of knowledge specifically in this area. Fourth, I have been given a referral to one such doctor in order to explore other options and possibilities for treatment. Fifth, having a hysterectomy is absolutely *not* an option for me. Sixth, I have about a month to wait before I can get in to be seen by this new doctor. Seventh, if I do nothing while I wait, chances are pretty high that the disease will continue to spread and things will get worse. Eight, however, if I at least continue with this new pain management regimen, in the meantime, there is also a chance that some of my symptoms will improve; if not, perhaps they won't progress either. Ninth, this new pain management drug (*Elavil*) might actually prove to be useful, since it is also used to treat depression, as well as chronic pain, and it just may keep me from spiraling out of control like I did before. Tenth, nothing left to do now, but watch, wait, and pray.

Friday, January 15th, 2010

I finally went to see that pelvic pain specialist and the good news is that she says I do not have to have a hysterectomy! Praise God for that! What she did say was that she thinks we should change my meds again. ☹ *Hopefully she will give me something that will control the pain, but not have me all loopy and sluggish like I am now. So I've got to take the current meds for one more week, then on this coming Friday, I will switch to the new stuff. It is good that I'm starting on the weekend; that way, if it does anything loopy to me, then I'll have the weekend to recover. Additionally both doctors recommended physical therapy with a pelvic floor specialist! They both agreed that with the [pelvic floor]therapist, it will help!*

Praise God! Thank you Jesus, Hallelujah and all that! My latest doctor, an Endo specialist said "You do not have to get a hysterectomy!" Those words washed over me with the refreshing coolness of a summer rain right in the middle of a hot sticky day! Talk about *waiting to exhale!* Whitney Houston didn't have anything on me! I don't think I ever sighed so deeply, so fully, so intentionally in all my life! When she said it, I wanted to leap off the exam table and kiss her! Instead I sat there as water filled my eyes with my hands cupped over my mouth. I was gasping "thank you" over- and-over again, while in my mind, I was channeling Sophia from **The Color Purple** thinking repeatedly: " *I knowed dere iz a Gawd!*"

Though I was not happy about changing medications again and having to go through another physical and emotional side effect/withdrawal adjustment, I was willing to try whatever it took in order to avoid being cut up, sliced and diced; especially if that meant it would bring me any measurable amount of relief. I had never heard of pelvic floor therapy before that day, but if it allowed me to keep my insides intact, I was willing to give it shot.

Feb 02, 2010

Sooooo, I'm changing meds again! This Neurontin crap has had me literally feeling like I'm on a roller coaster and I've been eating ravenously for damn near two weeks! And I am not having that. So, they're switching me back to the Elavil; this time at a significantly reduced dose! I do have to taper off this other crap for the next couple of days before I can do the switch. Hell, it was making me all loopy and it wasn't even controlling the pain! I'll be glad when I'm healed completely from this!

My uber excitement over not having to get a hysterectomy was slowly being replaced by the uncontrollable urge to punch somebody in the throat! And by somebody I meant the preverbal "mad scientists" who had since discovered a plethora ways to keep men sexually active until they are 100 years old, but could not come up with anything better for treating Endometriosis other than drug us or gut us! My resident frustration was becoming riled again! I truly could not understand it. Why was it so difficult to find a method of treatment or a plan that worked, continued to work, and work well? The doctors did not prepare me for this sh*t. I sincerely did not expect to still be dealing with this two years later! The constant cycle of: try this medication for two weeks, no switch to this one for a month, up this dose, lower that dose, see this specialist, try that therapist, take this test, get this scan, and wait for the results; it was beginning to make a *sistah* incredibly weary! I had laid on more beds and tables, flashed my privates to more strangers, and been poked, stuck, and stretched open by more cold, hard, metal objects than an X-rated porn star! I felt like a walking petri dish; A perpetual case study for some biological experiment! No wonder I ended up in therapy! It was taking all the determination I had for me not to end up back there again.

Sunday, March 21st, 2010

I'm a little nervous. I'm supposed to give myself a "break" from the continuous birth control starting tomorrow and I must admit

I'm not too thrilled about it. I have already been cramping most of the week. My right breast has been so swollen and my nipple is so tender, it's like my body knows what's coming! I could not have been ovulating, because everything was supposed to be shut down! I took three IB 800's with no apparent relief setting in. That was around 9 this morning, so, I just took a ½ norco to try to head off the major pain before it has a chance to set in. I mean REALLY set in. I've already had traces of blood in my urine for the past two days…so maybe the flow will start soon and end just as soon! The idea behind this whole "experiment", is that if I follow the "seasonique" method and take [the pill] for three months, then take a "break" and let my body have (or attempt to have) a period as a sort of a break – then I won't have these "episodes" where I bleed on and on for two and three months at a time. In theory, I can see how this would work. But in reality…I just don't know that it will.

July 16th, 2010

So, I went to the doc for my three month follow up since March. I'd had my second "period" (June) since then and had been doing okay. I was considering asking them to up my Elavil to 15mg, because it seems as if I've developed a tolerance to the 10mg. It just isn't controlling the pain as well as it used to. So just as I expected, they do a PAP smear. And when they go in they find something "funky looking" [their words not mine]on my cervix that doesn't look "quite right" [again, their words not mine]. So now, they have to go in and do some "extensive scraping" so that they can get a "really good" sample to see what's going on. Apparently some of the scar tissue on my cervix is or has been bleeding and that's usually where the bleeding comes from during sexual penetration or stimulation, [although not always the case]. So, in addition to all of that, I have to have another ultrasound done in October, after these test results come back and they have a better grasp of what's going on!

It seemed to me that they were always trying to get a better grasp of what was going on. As I sat there listening, it took all the God in me, to restrain myself from responding with the satirical line made famous by the character *Snoop* in the TV show *The Wire:* "Shiiiiiiiid, me too!"

2010

Exasperated sigh This is really frustrating, but I refuse to let it further discourage me. There's even talk of a biopsy to make sure it's not cancer, which I just rebuke right now in Jesus' name. They started throwing around that damned "H" word again– hyster-ectomy – which I also rebuke and refuse in Jesus' name as well! So, I'm just gonna wait and see, and in the meantime keep doing what I have to do.

CHAPTER 6
FIGHTING FIERCELY

"F*ck this, we 'bout to set it off"
~Queen Latifah as Cleo in Set It Off.

I didn't go into denial, I didn't go into depression, but I did get determined. I was determined not to be held hostage by this aggravating cycle of experimental treatments, followed by indefinite periods of hurrying up to wait. Being patient didn't mean being still; I had a life to live. I was a few weeks shy of my 35th birthday, almost four years into my journey as an entrepreneur; and while it hadn't been easy, I had made it through two years of an absolute living hell! It wasn't easy, but in spite of it all, I managed to: keep a small business thriving, my mental faculties intact, finally completed my home decorating project, and I had even managed to shed 30 pounds! I had a long way yet to go, but it was high time I started celebrating the long way I had already come. Acknowledgement was the first step in getting there and acceptance was the next. What better way to profess that acceptance than to strip down, bare all, and get honest and naked with myself…literally.

Choosing to do a nude photo shoot, at that particular time in my life was not only therapeutic, but incredibly symbolic for me in so many meaningful ways. On the surface, the physical correlation was clear. I would carry those surgical scars with me forever. Now, each time I saw myself, I would see them. Instead of being a reminder of something wretched and horrible every time I looked at them, they would now serve as a symbol of fortitude and triumph. They would now become a permanent reminder that I had overcome one of the most difficult trials and tests of my faith.

I spent the better part of the past two years being naked and exposed under circumstances that evoked a paralyzing sense of anxiety, apprehension, discomfort, embarrassment, awkwardness, and futility; this happened in an environment that was often stoic, unaffected, and hurtfully matter-of-fact. In contrast, I now needed to reclaim my nakedness in a way that would restore my sense of womanhood. I needed to see myself, remember myself, embrace

59

myself, in those imperative ways that would reestablish my softness, vulnerability, femininity; and yes, I'm just going to say it –

my sexiness!

July...

In preparation for this photo shoot, I was asked to write down all of the reasons why I decided to do this? Why do I want these images in the first place? I want these images because I will be turning 35 years old this year. For some reason this is such a significant time in my life as I have experienced such a tremendous amount of: change, triumph, tragedy, growth, maturity, and learning over the past two years. Physically, mentally, emotionally, professionally...there have been many, many hurdles! Part of my journey includes a 30 pound weight loss and I initially wanted to do the shoot to celebrate losing the physical weight, but as I thought more, I wanted to celebrate, not just the shedding of the pounds, but also the shedding of the guilt, shame, and embarrassment about my own body [and what this disease has done to it], my body image, my sexuality, sensuality, all those hang-ups about having the perfect body. I wanted to show acceptance of me and all my flaws, my imperfections, my scars, my stretch marks – all those things that I despised or wanted to hide about myself and my body. For some reason, as I approach 35, I've come to accept, embrace, and dare I say to love myself. Taking these photos would: first, show that I can actually stand to look at myself naked in the mirror; second, to be okay with what I see; and third, to look at the scars and be reminded that you've been through some battles, you may have some wounds, you many have some scars, but you are here! You made it through all of those things and you survived it! You are still here and better than before! As Ru Paul would say, "I am still FIIIII'ERCE!"

I needed to have that! When you go through an experience that significantly diminishes your ability or capacity to become a mother, or to control your reproductive planning on your own terms, which, for many of us, is one of the quintessential hallmarks of being: a woman, a wife, a girlfriend, or significant other, you feel lost. You feel: less than, unwanted, unloved, and without a purpose. That photo shoot helped me to take my self-love and purpose back.

August 21, 2010

Sooooo, I just got back from the photo shoot and I feel AMAZ-ING! Seph was so amazing and I felt so comfortable and beautiful and sexy and free...I was a little nervous, but I got comfortable right away. Even the rough drafts looked great and I even learned something about myself – I have a fabulous ass! It was weird at first seeing myself naked in print. But, the more I looked at the pictures, the more I fell in love with them; the more I fell in love with me and with God for allowing me to finally see myself the way He has always seen me! I am just on such a high right now! I still can't believe I did that, but I'm so glad that I did! Growth is a beautiful thang! It really truly is!

I kept my newfound momentum going for the rest of that year. I brought in 35 with a bang and I loved every minute of it! I threw a fabulous party where I reconnected with lots of family and friends, many of whom I had not seen, talked to, or spent time with since this whole sorted ordeal began. I drank, I danced, I laughed...with nary a hint of cramping or bleeding! I felt fantastic! I felt elated! I felt like....me!

As summer changed to fall, and fall gave way to winter, I felt like I had hit my stride. I had settled into the growing familiarity of my new routine, and I was living, loving, and breathing more freely. Over the next 15 months, though I would still have flare ups that would cause me to have to slow down at times, they were becoming much more scarce. My new medical team had finally secured a treatment regimen that was working exceptionally well for me. The combination of continuous birth control pills along with long term pain inhibitors (*Elavil*) was working wonders. The pelvic floor therapy was bringing incredible relief from the cramping. The inconvenience of having to endure occasional spotting or light "breakthrough bleeding" was a minuscule trade off that I was all too happy to give in exchange for not having to withstand the heinous atrocity that would otherwise be my monthly menstrual cycle. For the most part, I was down to one IB 800 a day, and my threshold for duration and intensity of physical and social activity continued to increase.

High heels and skinny jeans were making their way back into my wardrobe! Also, prints and colors, boy shorts , and thongs were back in the panty rotation! Now, for some of your reading this, underwear etiquette might not be a big deal to you, but, when you're in the throes of learning how to manage unpredictable, unexpected, uncontrollable Endo flares, **ALL** of your panties become "granny panties"! In fact, black cotton becomes the only real friend you have! So yes, after several months of being "flare-free", girlfriend threw herself a personal panty parade!

I still fought through self-induced fear mongering every time I went for my quarterly follow up's, but I refused to let the "what-ifs" cripple me. Fleeting anxieties aside, I started to approach my appointments with a more matter-of-fact attitude, instead of feeling like every visit was going to be a death sentence. I continued to learn as much as I could about Endometriosis. I studied many Endo-related websites and forums. Furthermore, I aligned myself with several online support communities. Being able to connect with Endo Sisters in other cities, states, and even countries, provided an incredible validation for everything I had encountered during my experience. Having other sisters share their stories with me confirmed that: I was not alone, I was not crazy, and this was not all in my head. Additionally, having them share their resources opened up a completely new world of information to me. My new discoveries empowered me to have greater control, while navigating this maze of uncertainty, when choosing treatment and management options for both my short and long term goals. I always kept my symptom journal close: documenting and notating, just in case.

November 2011

...Right at the end of the month, this stupid bleeding started – again! I was hoping that it would be some sort of fluke, but it wasn't...

December 2011

So, the bleeding continues and keeps getting worse...

January 2012

The specialist I was seeing in Evanston, didn't have any open-

ings until March, so, I scheduled something closer (at the hospital where I had my surgery). Since all of my original team was now gone, I had to choose someone from the directory. This dumb ass doctor totally dismissed the new symptoms I'm having which are really, really bad, on my right side! I really didn't want to think the worst, but I couldn't help but ponder if it's spreading to my right side and fucking up my right ovary and fallopian tube! Lord knows I think I would just die at the thought of not being able to have children naturally; although, now I'm starting to reconsider if I even want kids. With all the pain and agony I've been in, I don't even know if I would/could be a capable parent, even if I were to be able to get pregnant.

...I finally convinced this new doctor, after damn near having to "get black" on her ass, to schedule me a damned ultrasound to see what the f*ck is going on with this Endo. I told her, 'Look! I've already lost one ovary and tube to this and I don't want to continue to dismiss this and then it be too far gone by the time we (i.e. you and the rest of these dumb ass docs) finally figure out that something is wrong!' She still wasn't very supportive of it – she said – "Well I really do think it's because of [the fact that I missed a day taking] the pill, but I do think if it'll help to give you a peace of mind...we'll schedule it"... What the hell? I didn't care what the fuck she thought as long as I got my damned appointment!

I was pissed all the way off; And, egregiously insulted to say the least! I could not believe that I was sitting here having to debate with this doctor the validity and seriousness of what was going on inside my body! Here I was verbally sparring with this woman, trying to get her to at least consider the fact that I knew my own body well enough to discern that, after four years of living with and managing this monster, I knew that what was happening to me was not typical!

I'm not sure what hurt the most: her cold, uninterested display of nonchalance and indifference, or the fact that this brazen, dismissive attitude was being tossed in my face by a doctor who was a woman.

The fact that she was a woman of color made the sting even more palpable! In my experience, when it comes to issues having to do with all things *ladyparts*, one would presume to expect a certain degree of detachment from any men that you might encounter, including doctors (the biggest reason being that because of the obvious differences, men would not be able to relate to the delicate nature surrounding, well, our delicate nature). But when dealing with a woman, I just assumed I would be met with an outpouring of empathy and understanding; an overwhelming desire to help me put an end to yet another *winter of discontent*.[33] I learned that day why Lauryn Hill once said that, "expectation is the mother of all disappointment."

She kept insisting that all of this was happening to me as a result of me possibly missing a birth control pill or two over the past couple of months! It took all the home training my parents instilled in me, for me not to reach across that desk and claw her vacant eyes out! Instead, I clasped my hands together, placed them in my lap, leaned forward very cautiously, looked directly and piercingly into her eyes, taking great care to enunciate with as much clarity and firmness as I could muster, and I told her with a very measured and even tone: *"Lady, I could have missed an entire pack of birth control pills and I would not be bleeding like this! I have been bleeding continuously since November! SOMETHING-IS-WRONG-WITH-ME!"*

When I returned for the results of the ultrasound a few days later, as she walked into the room, she couldn't even look me in the face. Looking at her not looking at me, my heart sank. Sliding into the chair behind her desk, and placing the documents that undoubtedly told the tale on top, she gazed up at me rather sheepishly and said: "It's bad. It's really bad."

She then proceeded to go on and on about how sorry she was and how Endo wasn't really her specialty. Her best recommendations for me was to either: have a hysterectomy or to get pregnant as soon as possible. As if her advice wasn't insulting enough, she only made matters worse when she said "You know you're running out of time. What are you waiting for anyway?"

I wanted to tell her that what I had been waiting for was a more consistent quality of care in my treatment. I had been waiting to be taken seriously from the onset by dismissive doctors exactly like her. I had been waiting to have my needs and concerns fully understood and addressed. What I had been waiting for was my mind to get my emotions under control before I relented to my impulse to reach across the table and slap her face!

Instead, I simply told her: *"Weeeeelll* for one, while there are lots of things that I can do by myself, getting pregnant is not one of them. And, I'd really like to be married first. I'm not really interested in becoming a *baby mamma* on purpose."

And just when I thought the disrespect couldn't get any worse, she proceeds to give me unsolicited dating advice by telling me: "Well, technically you know you *couuuuuld* get pregnant by yourself. And, while you out there looking for a husband…" She paused and looked around, leaning in intently. Then, in an epic fail of an attempt at some sort of secret, *sistah-girl* bonding moment, spat out, "…you *know* he ain't gotta be black."

BLANKSTARE *CRICKETS* *RAPIDLY BLINKING EYES*

Time stopped! Did she *really* just say that to me? You could have stuck a fork in me right then and there because I was absolutely D-O-N-E! Had she stopped chuckling long enough to read my reaction, she might have had enough time to deflect the daggers I was throwing at her with my eyes.

She further went on to recommend me to yet another doctor; this time, a colleague who supposedly had more expertise in "this area." After hearing what I had just heard her say to me, I had absolutely no confidence in anybody that she might recommend. But, what could I do? It would still be several more weeks before I could get in to see my own specialist, and I could not bear to go that long doing absolutely nothing. Besides, it wasn't really fair to hold the abysmal ignorance of this one individual against someone I'd never met before. If my Endo had come back as aggressively as she'd alluded to, and if my options for remedy were as narrow as the only two she had given me, I was going to be sure to visit as many specialists and get as many second opinions as I needed in order for me to make the most informed decision possible. I could at least hear what he had to say.

Early March 2012,

*I spent most of the month depressed, still bleeding and shuffling form doctor-to-doctor trying to figure out what the hell is wrong with me. Because they found that my Endo had spread inside my uterus, I had now been diagnosed with a second condition called **adenomyosis** . There was also significant irritation, and inflammation in my fallopian tube, to the point where, they initially thought it was going to rupture! Of course I was losing my mind, because all this was occurring on my right side, which is now, my only viable side that would allow me to conceive since of course they have removed everything from my left side. Then, to drive me even more crazy, they started talking about rupturing tubes, removing tubes, harvesting, freezing and storing eggs, IVF, surrogates and all kinds of crazy sh*t.....*

I seriously thought my head was going to explode! Charlie Brown's teacher was back with a vengeance! And rambling with such rapid spitfire, I instantly caught a migraine. Before I could even attempt to process everything that was being thrown at me, assistants were hovering overhead, offering to get me scheduled for my hysterectomy "as early as next week." WHAT THE F*CK WAS WRONG WITH THESE PEOPLE! WHAT DIDN'T THEY UNDERSTAND ABOUT MY RIGHT, MY CHOICE, MY DECLARATION THAT GETTING A HYSTERECTOMY WAS A NON-F*CKING-FACTOR FOR ME! IT WAS NOT AN OPTION TO BE CONSIDERED!! Why didn't these people get it? If I had learned enough in my own investigations to comprehend the fact that having a hysterectomy was NOT a definitive cure for endometriosis, then why couldn't these "professionals" get that through their thick skulls! What did I need to do? Get "NO HYSERECTOMY" tattooed across my forehead AND my vagina? Or was I going to have to jump up on the desk, smack my lips, roll my eyes, prop my one hand on my hips, while giving him the *"don't go there'"* stance with the other. Was I going to have to charismatically conjure up the character *New-New* from the movie *ATL* and let them know with an emphatic southern drawl, just as she had: *"UHNN UH, NOT.GON. HAPPEN!"*

As they buzzed about grabbing pamphlets and consent forms and pulling up electronic calendars, I stood up, and gathered my things. I wiped my tear stained face and promptly told them that

I would not be scheduling any surgeries that day. I needed time to absorb these new developments and weigh my options. They were not going to dictate to me my next steps. Rather, I would let them know, when I was ready, what I would choose as my final decision.

Remembering the coping skills that I'd gained in therapy, I left that hospital with a completely different attitude. I wasn't sad, I wasn't angry, and I wasn't depressed. I was, however, even more determined. I was not about to let my fate be handed to me without fighting with all that I had to have the final say. When I got home, I immediately plugged in to several of my online support groups. I told the ladies about my latest ordeal and asked if any of the local sisters or medical experts on the forum could provide me with any recommendations for Endo specialists in the area. As it turned out, there were several. One in particular, whose office was located in Skokie, IL, just happened to be the partner of the specialist that I was on the waiting list to see. I thought to myself, *"what the hell?"* If they were a part of the same medical team, there was a pretty good chance that he'd be just as good as she was, if not better. Something had to give. I refused to keep being tossed to-and-fro, from doctors office to doctors office, only to come up more empty than before. I prayed to God that he was available, and that somehow, he would be able to help me. I was starting to feel the steadfast resolve that I had spent the last two years building slowly start to chip away from under me. I could not let that happen. God must have been listening, because, he was able to see me just three days after I called for an appointment.

After reviewing my history, and all the reports I had forwarded over from the other doctors, he confirmed that, in fact, the Endo had spread and had developed into adenomyosis. He had also confirmed the swelling and fluid buildup in my right fallopian tube. To my dismay, he also surmised there was the possibility that the tube may have to be taken out, but he had rather not jump into another surgery right away if there was no urgent need. There were a few less invasive alternatives that he had that he wanted to explore first.

Luckily I've found a very progressive doctor who wanted to try a wait and see approach first, before yanking my insides straight the f*ck out! His priority was to get my bleeding under control and stop the pain first. He said that my fallopian tube was not in immediate danger of rupturing and that sometimes the fluid will subside on its own. He said that he's seen worse cases that had a complete turnaround [without requiring surgery]. So, I agreed to wait and see.

While the wait and see approach was not entirely new to me, I was more accepting of it this time around, because, we actually had a plan in place: a very definitive plan. We were monitoring for very specific outcomes, with particular courses of action in place that would be dependent upon those outcomes. And, this was an approach that had been proven successful with past patients. That is what made me comfortable. That is what made me trust him. That is what made me confident that I still had a stake in this fight!

There's a story that my cousin Gwen once told me about the revelation that my Grandmother offered when asked how she knew that my Grandfather was, "The One." As the story goes, when asked the question, my Grandmother pondered in silence for a few moments, after which she glanced up, looked over at my cousin with a certain reflectiveness and answered, very simply and assuredly:

"Well, I just decided...."

On the bus ride back from Skokie that afternoon, my Grandmother's assertion played over-and-over in my mind. Now battling my third relapse with this disease, I finally got it. When it came to something so important, so affecting, so life changing for my grandmother, she simply made a decision. It was time for me to make a decision too.

By the time I made it home that afternoon, I had decided that I had enough. I was done being afraid. I was done being ashamed. I was done being held hostage by this *thing* that had the professionals just as confused and dumbfounded as those of us suffering with it. I decided that if I had to live with this anomaly that was affecting my life to such an astounding degree that I was going to do just that: L-I-V-E! I didn't know what I was going to do, but I had to do something!

When I was first diagnosed, I thought Endometriosis was a recent epidemic. It left me absolutely dumbstruck to know that this disease had been running rampant underground for decades and yet so very little was known about its pathology and effects. I asked myself, If I had muddled my way through the past four years feeling confused, alone, and downright crazy, how many other women were feeling the same way? If I had spent the last 20 years erroneously believing that debilitating pain, uncontrollable cramps, copious and continuous bleeding was normal, and even an expected rite of passage on the road to "womanhood", how many young girls were being fed this same bowl of ignorance right now? Why didn't more people know about this disease? Why weren't people talking about this anomaly? Why weren't there commercials about diagnosis and treatment? Why weren't there Endo brochures in the doctors' offices alongside the ones for: PAP Smears, Mammograms, and STD prevention? Why wasn't this part of the national conversation as it relates to women's reproductive and gynecological health and wellbeing?

March 2012

So, with the epiphany of this third bout with this crazy disease, I really felt pressed in my Spirit to do something. I decided to throw an awareness event to bring light to this horrible disease and the many woman, children, and even girls (as young as 11) who are affected by it. Many of them being women of color.

The next week I went to work! I scoured my rolodex, and reached out to many of my contacts in my entrepreneurial and business networks. I talked to my doctors. I also talked to the educational program director at the Endometriosis Association. Before I knew it, along with the help of some tremendously supportive friends, family, and business partners, I had assembled a two day event featuring a line-up of: medical experts, nutritionists, physical therapists, and Endo-survivors (including myself). All these parties were coming together to: educate, enlighten, and empower the public about this crippling phenomenon that has been adversely affecting millions of women every year. Yet, unless you were one of these women, no one seemed to even know about it.

On that day, my *Fighting Fiercely*™ awareness campaign for Endometriosis was born!

...So, I got on my P's and Q's, started praying and doing a lot of research, reached out...and in the end, it came together really nicely...I was able to get sponsors for the photos, video, decorations, snacks, and speakers. It was really awesome and though I was nervous at first, I'm really glad I ended up letting God use me! I really felt good about doing it and I figured, as cliché as it sounds, if I was able to help just ONE person get diagnosed or find new or different ways to get relief from her symptoms, or to be able to lend support for a woman who is suicidal like I was, the I truly did my job. The event was called, Fighting Fiercely for YOU: An Endometriosis Awareness Event. It went over so well, I think I'm going to do it again next year!

Fighting Fiercely™ was the first time I ever shared my entire story publicly. Over the years, I had shared bits and pieces with a friend or two, but never with the degree of transparency that I shared at this event. I didn't do it for recognition. I didn't do it for the spotlight, I didn't do it for any accolades. I did it because over the past four years I had done a tremendous amount of hurting. I spent a great deal of time feeling confused and alone. For the longest time, I wanted nothing more than to take everything I had experienced in the past 48 months and bury it so far, so deep, in a place where nobody would ever find it, and I would never have to deal with it again! But after my third ride on this Endo roller coaster, I realized that was not going to happen. It wasn't supposed to happen. That was not part of His plan. I did not know why I had to be the one, I certainly did not ask to be the one. As private a person as I am by nature, I certainly did not want to be the one. But, as long as there were other women out there long suffering in silence, feeling as confused and alone as I had felt, then I had to do something. If I could give a voice to their story by sharing my own, if my mess of a life over the past four years could result in a message that would inspire, encourage, and support women in letting them know that they too could, in fact, L-I-V-E with this disease, and live life more abundantly, then I would gladly answer the call.

Fight - verb (used without object), fought, fight·ing.

to engage in battle or in single combat; attempt to defend one-self against or to subdue, defeat, or destroy an adversary. [34]

Fierce(ly) – adj, wild or turbulent in force, action, or intensity; vehement, intense, or strong: fierce competition. [35]

being bold, displaying chutzpah, especially relating to fashion, clothes, hair or makeup. [36]

In March of 2014, my *Fighting Fiercely*™ campaign celebrated its third year of raising awareness in support of Endometriosis. As long as Endometriosis exists, and until a cure is found, I will continue to do my part no matter how big or small, to: educate, enlighten, and empower sufferers, survivors, and supporters of any woman stricken with this awful, horrible, terrible disease. And I will continue to fight FIERCELY!

CHAPTER 7
ALL IN THE FAMILY

"It's a family afaiiiiir" Sly & The Family Stone.

It has been emphatically stated by numerous *experts* that Endometriosis is not really, a *life threating* disease. Please allow me to challenge the entire *status quo* on that theory. My goal is to boldly dispute that claim as complete B.S. and here's why:

First, let's take a look at that term, life-threatening in a bit more detail. Generally speaking, this term has often been used for describing something that is known to be an eminent cause or has a direct correlation thereby resulting in death. However, I would like to challenge you: just because Endometriosis doesn't cause death the way a bullet to the brain might, it certainly demands an alternate perception of the concept. While a woman may not die from the pathology of endometriosis, she will most always experience a death in varying degrees to her quality of life.

According to the World English Dictionary (2014), life and threat can be defined as:

Life - n, a present condition, state, or mode of existence. [37]

Threat - n, a person or thing that is regarded as dangerous or likely to inflict pain or misery. [38]

Endometriosis is more than *likely* to inflict pain, that is exactly what it does. Even for women who do not experience significant levels of physical pain with Endo, the emotional and psychological trauma can take a devastating toll. Misery is one of the most common feelings associated with the ramifications of this disease. At the time of this writing, it has been reported, based on awareness and advocacy activities in several of my online support groups in the Endo community, that eight women have taken their lives due to the feelings of hopeless and helplessness that can be brought on by dealing with this disease.

In my opinion, to say that endometriosis is not life threating is as dangerous as the use of the word in its very definition.

The U.S. National Library of Medicine (2011) confirms that:

> More severe forms of endometriosis could affect nearly every area of a woman's life. Many feel less womanly. Particularly young women with strong symptoms may not be able to develop a positive relationship to their own body. Painful sex can make it difficult to have an enjoyable sex life. Women who have more serious forms of endometriosis might not be able to become pregnant and have their own children. Chronic pain may lead to depression, tiredness and irritability. Together, all of these factors can place a heavy burden on a relationship.[39]

Again, I challenge *powers that be* to digest the information presented in the above quote and yet continue to assert that endometriosis is not life threatening. The chronic pain, fertility concerns, and potentially negative impact on a woman's body image and self-esteem can absolutely threaten her quality of life. The article goes on to state that:

> For a considerable number of women, the recurring pain means that their everyday lives are repeatedly "disrupted" because they are unable to carry out their usual activities, go to work or pursue their hobbies. Women who cannot go to work due to their pains and cramps often face feelings of guilt and shame. [40]

Not only is the core of a woman's physical essence jeopardized by endometriosis, but her professional life, social life, and emotional stability is challenged as well. When a woman is overwrought by guilt and shame, (often projected onto her by others) because of this disease, all areas of her life can swiftly sink into a dangerous state of being. Sadly, some women unwittingly cross that delicate threshold of becoming a danger to themselves.

The Endometriosis Association (2010) reports: "While some women's lives are relatively unaffected by it, too many others have suffered with severe pain, emotional stress, have at times been unable to work, or carry on normal activities, and have experienced financial and relationship problems because of the disease." [41]

If the aforementioned consequences are not such that impose vast amounts of pain, misery, or danger to a woman's present condition, state, or mode of existence, then perhaps we need to redefine *threat*, because I don't know many other circumstances that warrant such a caution.

Endometriosis not only impacts the women afflicted with it, the damaging effects often ripple out, to impact: personal, professional, social, romantic, and nearly all the lives of those closest to us. The physical, mental, and emotional struggles associated with endometriosis have been known to cause, sometimes irreparable damage, to some of our most cherished relationships.

"The Men All Pause" ~Klymaxx.

March 2009

I've met someone. Yeah, yeah, I know...I know.

The first time I had to tell a guy about my Endo, it really wasn't by choice. We had fallen into a nightly routine of chatting with each other every night before bedtime (which always happened to be right around the time when my evening dose of meds would start to kick in). Without realizing it, I would find myself: nodding off in the middle my sentences and losing my train of thought right at the heart of a conversation. If that wasn't embarrassing enough, I would sometimes uncontrollably slur my words. Of course, I wasn't aware of any of this, until he kindly brought it to my attention. At that point, the "jig was up"! I couldn't keep running from the inevitable. I paused, took a deep breath, and let it all out. I was compelled to tell him the good, the bad, and the ugly about everything I'd gone through over the past year. His response was not what I expected. He said, *"oh, so that's why you talk so slow and sexy to me every night...it's the meds...hmmm, medicated sexy – I think I like it."* From then on, that became one of his "pet names" for me, *medicated sexy.* Sure, it was a little corny, but I appreciated his attempt to connect what I was going through with something positive and romantic. His compassion even helped me handle my subsequent Endo flares with a little more grace and dignity.

Many Endo women are not as blessed as I had been in that regard. As a matter of fact, I wasn't as lucky the next time around.

The second time I attempted to foray into dating (post-Endo), the conversation did not go as smoothly as I had planned it in my head. I really liked this new guy. I mean, I really liked this guy, so much so, that every time I was around him: I got the butterflies in my stomach, I was nervous, jittery, always blushing, everything you'd expect with a new romance. Because I had such a good experience before, I figured this time around, I would be proactive in my policy of disclosure. I wanted to be honest with him before my *"medicated sexy"* gave him the wrong idea. The problem was, my perfectly planned dissertation constantly got lost in translation on its way from my brain to my mouth. In reality, I always found myself stumbling all over my thoughts and words…falling right into the realm of embarrassment that I had been so desperately trying to avoid. I seriously doubt that he ever did grasp the fullness of what I was trying to convey. As a result: my mood swings, my overtly emotional sensitivity, and the intensity of my pain spikes were completely lost on him. I was just not able to express myself in the same way that I had with the previous guy, so the relationship essentially fell apart before it even got started.

For many women with Endo, romantic relationships can be a very intimidating, anxiety filled course that is not always easy to navigate. The typical complexities involved in forming and maintaining intimate relationships, whether it be in the context of dating or marriage, are often exacerbated when endometriosis is added to the equation. Many Endo Sisters have shared their similar story countless times. It can be a very painful experience to have a boyfriend leave or a husband file for divorce, all because they may have a lack of understanding, an inability to know how to help, or when the disruption of intimacy (e.g. no sex) becomes entirely too much for them to handle.

Because an Endo flare can strike at any time, with varying degrees of intensity, the seemingly simple act of just going on a date can become a huge gamble. We have to worry about: if/when we are going to start bleeding, is it going to soak though our clothes while we're out, will we make it through the date before needing to take a pain pill, and/or if we were to take a pain pill beforehand, how long we would have before we experienced the marked drowsiness and slurred speech. Additionally, did we even: bring enough pads, pills, or an extra set of panties in case we needed to make an emergency trip to the bathroom? Having all of those worries at the same time, can make one a tad bit unfocused on a date. Simply contemplating when-or-how to even bring up the topic of endometriosis to a potential suitor is not an exciting task to have to consider. It will be awkward no matter when we do it, and let's face it- it is not the most stimulating topic of conversation.

For women who are in married or committed relationships, the difficulties do not end there. With all of the traumatic activity that goes on in-and-around the vagina, many women can become very guarded and protective of that area. Also, many of the activities that used to be a source of love, pleasure, and connectedness with their partners, can often disintegrate into a source of dread, hopelessness, and even helplessness.

A woman's sexual prowess, along with her sexual self-esteem, can be severely hampered by endometriosis; especially, if she has been subjected to multiple surgeries and hormonal treatments. Oftentimes because of what is happening on the inside, a woman can feel absolutely ugly on the outside. A woman may have trouble finding herself sexually appealing and may adamantly reject the notion that her partner will be sexually attracted to her. In addition, layering the bed with oversized beach towels, least we get startled by spontaneous "spills" in the middle of the night, and taking pre-emptive doses of pain medications to try to ward off cramps before they start, hardly makes for intriguing foreplay. In fact, it's all but guaranteed to dull the prospect of a free spirited *quickie* in the middle of the night!

Sometimes we are simply physically unable to perform. Rather than taking the embarrassing risk of not being able to satisfy our mates, the shame may subconsciously show up in the guise of: pushing them away, starting an argument, or not being in the mood – again!

From a sexual perspective, Endometriosis can trigger mood swings, heightened emotions, physical pain of penetration, inability to orgasm, or fear of orgasm because of the overwhelming pain or unexpected rush of blood that might accompany the *Big O*. Speaking of which, it is rather difficult to enjoy the experience when you are panicked about what sudden *surprises* may pour out, if your mate is one who enjoys certain... *oral* indulgences (yes, I'm talking about exactly what you think I'm talking about). All of these things terrify us and most days it's just easier to withdraw rather than to feel like a burden to your partner or the relationship. It weighs incredibly heavy on our hearts when we have to grapple with choosing between enjoying our mate for a few hours a night verses enduring the betrayal of our bodies for several days, weeks, or possibly months thereafter.

Men please hear, understand, and know: we are just as frustrated, aggravated and bewildered as you are. We want to be close to you, we want to express our love and appreciation for you in those very special, sacred, intimate, and passionate ways. Yes, we absolutely *"wanna put that thannnng on ya!"* But sometimes...... we simply can't.

In chatting with many of my Endo Sisters over the years, I have found that the issue of sexual intimacy, is one we find ourselves discussing often. The frustration, and lack of understanding repeatedly heaped upon us by our mates, only adds to the weight of guilt and embarrassment that we already carry. Many times, in our talks, we find that we share many of the same heartbreaking sentiments, such as:

"My husband is just fed up of Endo affecting our lives, like sex for one. It's just so hard to bottle up feelings of pain, guilt and total isolation due to Endo. I often tell him to find someone else! He should have a wife that can do normal things and have a sex life, instead of stoned on strong pain medication, heat pads, etc. Then again, I don't deserve to be ignored and feel uncared for either. It's so hard on a couple at times." ~ Sarah W.

"... Relationships are difficult. I never realized until last year when I got diagnosed that I had Endometriosis. With the laps and excision I had done, it now hurts to have intimacy. I never used to have a problem, in fact it helped my cramps... It is a daily struggle, but we just live the best that we can. It is awful that they do not have much to offer us women with Endo besides surgeries and hormones." ~ Stephanie D.

"The biggest obstacle to my relationships has been learning to believe that I really deserve love despite my flaws, both the physical and emotional ones."~ Michelle N.

"I've heard other women say that their boyfriend or husband have told them "Just take plenty of pain meds. to numb you or drink enough to numb you so we can have sex for more than a little time...so we can go longer and do different positions...I'll let you sleep afterwards!" That sickens me to no end. She wants to make love too...don't pressure her into it!" ~ Peggy Von Wyden

Men, imagine for just a moment that shocked, intense, and stabbing pain that would suddenly overtake you if accidentally got kicked in your testes. And let's say, for the sake of illustration, that this accidental injury caused them to swell to about twice their normal size. Because of your injury you now start bleeding from the tip of your penis and you keep bleeding. Now imagine that it alternates between a slow annoying drip and a constant stream. You feel as if you are urinating on yourself. This goes on for days at a time. Imagine you are not sure of the cause, so you call to make an appointment with your doctor. Imagine that it will be weeks before you will be seen. In the meantime, you pick up a box of *depends* to help prevent ruining your clothes during your daily activities. You have no idea when the incessant bleeding will stop.

Think about the inconvenience and embarrassment that starts to take its toll, but you try to put on a good game face for: your mate, your family and your friends. You attempt to go on with business as usual, but you find yourself increasingly fatigued due to the anemia. Just when you think things could not get any worse, metaphorically, a small herd of horses decide to bring their miraculous 24-hour tap dancing show right to the middle of your sacrum. They take up residence for an indefinite engagement! Add to that the random rectal spasms. Any semblance of your personal comfort has all but evaporated.

Nevertheless, you are still expected to give 100% of yourself at work, come home, pick up the kids from practice, mow the lawn, take out the trash, rub your honey's feet, and finish the home improvement project that you've been promising to get to for the past six months. You have to do all of this while you're still: bleeding, having spasms, and looking for relief for your swollen, uncomfortable, now chaffed testes(from all the constant rubbing against the *Depends*) and incessantly bleeding penis. Now, imagine that you finally get to see your doctor and he blatantly informs you that while there is no cure for what's wrong with you, you can opt to have a surgery that requires all sorts of instruments to be inserted into that little tiny hole at the tip of your penis. He also tells you that it might be necessary to remove one or of both your testicles. And finally, he matter-of-factly forewarns you that the procedure will likely result in the loss of two or more inches from the length of your penis, along with some relatively gruesome scarring, which by the way, may or may not bring you relief from your symptoms- Perhaps. Possibly. Maybe. However, they cannot make any guarantees.

Now, having let the shock and awe of that marinate with you for a while, you finally schlep your way home from the doctor's office, and collapse onto the sofa. As you sit there, you try to figure out a way to drop this spectacular bit of news on your woman, especially after last week's conversation about trying one more time to get that baby girl in a house full of three boys. Imagine, she softly emerges from the bedroom and seductively slides in close to you on the sofa. She peers over, sizing you up with that "knowing" look in her eyes. Leaning in close, she whispers in your ear, as my Daddy has been known to say to his wife… *"Pardon me, but ummm, you think I could get a lil' bit of your time this evening?"*

PAUSE. Men, take a moment, to absorb what you just read. Immerse yourself in that situation for a moment to: see it, feel it, and listen to it. Can you imagine this scenario wreaking havoc on your emotions? Is your manhood being challenged? How attractive, capable, or worthy are you feeling in this moment?

What you have just imagined is what every Endo Woman has experienced at least once in her journey.

Remember, when you are in a relationship with an Endo Woman, the last thing she needs after being dismissed by the doctors, pharmacists, supervisors at work, and medical "experts", is to be dismissed by the one person who is supposed to be her strength when she is, literally, too weak to stand for herself. The most important things that we do need from you are: patience, understanding, and empathy – NOT sympathy – we don't need you to feel sorry for us. What we need is for you to at least make an attempt to connect with our experience in a: sincere, loving and supportive way.

Nothing hurts more or adds more depth to the pain we feel, than being berated with such remarks as:

"Dayum girl, you bleeding again!"

"You STILL bleeding?"

"Didn't you just HAVE a period?"

"You just being lazy, ain't nobody hurtin' THAT bad."

"All women get cramps, get over it."

"Can't you just take some *Tylenol?*"

"You're just using this as an excuse!"

"Great, so now we have to cancel _____ AGAIN!"

"Well, when is it gonna stop?"

"I'm a MAN, I got needs!"

"Soooooo, you just gon' lay in the bed all day? You not gonna cook or clean or deal with the kids?"

"You just don't wanna gimmie none."

"Well…. why can't we just do that *'other thing'?*"

"You just f*ckin' somebody else."

"I can't take this anymore, It's OVER!"

As women, we naturally look to our partners to be our rock and even more so when we're dealing with Endometriosis. We need you to be our cornerstone of support, not a boulder to crush us and break us down. Endo does that to us enough.

The lack of intimacy can be one of the most frustrating aspects of being in relationship with an Endo Woman. To be completely honest, there will be times when you just simply won't be able to *"do the do"*...at least not the "good ol' fashioned" way. Don't let that discourage you. Use those times as an opportunity to love outside the box by engaging in more sensual, though not necessarily sexual forms of intimacy such as: kissing, cuddling, caressing, or even simply holding, which can be a very small act that can go a long way in making her feel loved and secure. Try taking a sensual dance class, a couples massage class, or even a cooking class together; It could be one that highlights preparing dishes and desserts that double as aphrodisiacs.

For a fun and flirty experience, you can also try visiting an adult intimacy store. Believe it or not, many of these stores offer educational workshops and seminars on a variety of topics relating to keeping the intimacy going in the midst of medical challenges. Some have interesting lines of physical supports, pillows, and cushions to assist with positioning. There are manuals and books that can even offer guidance. My favorite store, *Early 2 Bed* here in Chicago, has an exclusive line of products that are specifically designed to help strengthen the pelvic floor and minimize pelvic pain with sexual intimacy – a challenging dilemma faced by most Endo Women.

Men, if you notice that her demeanor is particularly sluggish or you know that she is in the middle of a flare up, this is your cue to step up- and-step in to help. You can: wash/fold the laundry, order a pizza for dinner, arrange the play dates for the kids, put the kids to bed, run her a bath, make her a nice hot cup of tea, or even show her you care by gently caressing her stomach. In addition, help her by making sure that all of her "supplies' are within reach. Be comforting, encouraging, soft, gentle, and most of all, be patient.

If you're interested in a man's perspective on how to support an Endo Woman, The Good Men Project (2013) has an excellent article written by Pete Biesner entitled: **"23 Tips For Men on Supporting a Partner with Chronic Pain."** [42] What I love most about this article, is that he breaks down the tips into two categories, "The first set of tips is for supporting someone you love who has chronic pain. The second set of tips are practical suggestions for how to support a woman in an episode of critical pain..." [43]

The second set of tips that Bisner references can also be applicable to us when we're in the acute throes of an Endo flare. Although Biesner (2013) speaks from the relationship perspective of husband and wife, these tips will be useful for any stage of relationship with an Endo Woman:

Figure 4:

Tips For Men
on Supporting a Partner with Chronic Pain

I think that it is important to think of pain as your common enemy, not as a part of your wife or baggage that comes with her. It is something outside of both of you that impacts both of you and that can kill your marriage.

If your wife is anything like mine, she will try to hide her pain from you. She does it for two reasons: one, she does not want to be a wuss or a whiner. Second, she knows that her in pain is distressing for those that she loves, so she hides it from us.

To avoid a pain-storm, be on the look-out for non-verbal clues of increased pain. My wife who is normally a font of cheerful patter gets quieter the further into pain that she goes because she does not want her voice to betray her pain. She holds her body more rigid, trying not to limp and holds her breath, taking one long rasping breath for every three that I take. There is also a look of grim determination that settles in her eyes, even if she is smiling

Chronic pain does not mean that the person has the same level of pain every day or even at various times in the day. So encourage her to put the fun stuff first. If she has enough energy and pain relief to do a quick trip out and about, encourage her to go someplace fun rather than the grocery store

83

Don't let her "should" on herself—beat herself up for what she cannot do. Argue back when she expresses guilt or sets impossible expectations for herself. When my wife tells me that she is a bad mother because she couldn't stand in the rain beside a soccer field, I remind her of all the other ways that she has been there for our kids. Encourage her to tell significant people in her life such as her boss and co-worker that her life is significantly impacted by pain. Remind her that stating the truth is not the same as complaining and it does not make her a whiner.

One of my early ways of dealing with my wife's chronic pain was to encourage my wife not to do things that caused her pain. Then I realized that if she avoided all activities that caused her pain, she would never do anything. Let her grit her teeth and get through pain for things that are important to her, even if it kills you to watch her do it. And trust your wife if she says that she wants to have sex even while in pain. Sometimes and in some women, arousal can do wonders to offer temporary relief from pain.

Control access to your wife based on your wife's wishes, and especially her level of introversion or extroversion. My best friend's wife is a social butterfly. So when she recently had a mastectomy, she wanted everyone there. When my wife is in pain, she doesn't even want her own mother in the room. She wants me, a firmly closed door and darkened room. My job is to not allow her to guilt herself into allowing visitors when she is not up to it. Here is the tricky thing: If you are new to the relationship or if you haven't been that close lately, your wife may want someone else's care. It sucks, but suck it up and be there for her in whatever way she will allow.[44]

The tips listed here (figure 4) are a great place to start, particularly if you've never been in a relationship with a woman who lives with chronic pain. You can view the complete list in its entirety by visiting the website www.goodmenproject.com. [45]

If you are in relationship with an Endo Woman, and if you do not know anything about Endometriosis, then you need to get educated. Start by researching the topic for yourself. Ask questions! Accompany her on her doctor's visits. Offer to sit in on one of her support groups. Seek out Endo support groups and resources specifically for men. Talk to her! When you are finished, you should talk to her some more. Most of all, LISTEN, and respond accordingly.

I think that Biesner (2013) does an excellent job of contextualizing our plight, while conveying a relatable sense of empathy for the woman that he loves. He brilliantly ties it all together when he states:

> Trust me when I say that you do not want to be surprised by your wife's pain. The wall of pain will hit her hard, and if you are lucky she will end up snapping at your or the kids. If you are unlucky, she will collapse into sobs that will break your heart to hear…There is nothing that makes me feel as helpless as watching my wife suffer. I would far rather just absorb the pain myself…But I have discovered that while going away physically or emotionally may be less painful for me, it is selfish and actually adds to my wife's suffering. Being strong for her does not mean hiding my feelings…All that being a husband and a good man requires that I stay by her side in body, mind and heart and that I do what is within my power to ease her pain, offer her comfort and support her. [46]

I sincerely believe that any man reading this, who is willing to open himself up and take Biesner's tips to heart, will inevitably find that, while your conventional sense of relationship etiquette may be challenged, and while you may have to cast aside traditional dating notions and establish you own unique sense of normal, it is more than possible to have a loving, nurturing, and fulfilling relationship with a women who has Endometriosis.

"Where my girls at?" ~702.

I can still remember the confused look on my friends face when I told her for the *umpteenth* time during the summer following my surgery, that I would not be able to hang out because of complications with Endo. *"But, you had your surgery, right? So, you're okay now…right?"* Sighing deeply, I tried to explain to her as best I could, how the surgery didn't "fix" everything, and how there is not currently a cure. I tried my best to paint a picture that would illustrate for her the nature of a "flare up" and how that tremendously affected my ability to physically and emotionally participate in many of the activities that we were used to doing together. When I finally finished my explanation, she just looked up, shook her head and replied, *"Dayum, 'Chelle, that's messed up."*

Your romantic and intimate relationships aren't the only ones that are affected when you're dealing with Endometriosis. Next to your mate, the relationships with your girlfriends are some of the closest ones you can have. Sometimes, they can be even closer than family.

Throughout my journey: from my first ER visit, to after my surgery, and during my initial recovery period, several of my closest girls rallied around me like the true friends I knew they were. For example, When I was in the hospital, Tasha brought me flowers and braided my hair. Tracee would sneak in and stay past visiting hours just to keep me company. On my last day there, Boogie walked me back-and-forth across my hospital room, and fed me warm water and hot tea until my stomach settled. She waited until I passed that customary "poop" the doctors need to see before they would release you. When I got home, my "bestie" since the second grade, Daphne, brought me groceries. My amazing cousin Gwen, a fellow Endo Sister herself, drove all the way from Minnesota to help: clean house, walk me back-and-forth to the bathroom, listen to me (during my half-awake/half asleep induced slurred speech,panic filled rants), and lend her shoulder for my incoherent slobbering and uncontrollable crying spells. Having these friends (Tasha, Tracee, Boogie, Daphne, and Gwen) there for me during those critical first days meant absolutely everything to me.

As I progressed in my external recovery, much like everyone else, my friends thought that I was just fine. When summer hit, they were all excited for me to fall back into our routine of doing all things: festivals, concerts, movies, and restaurants! I hated seeing the disappointed looks in their eyes and hearing the sullen tone of their voices week-after-week when I had to tell them: *"Nahhh girl, I won't be able to make it"* or *"I would love to go, but I'm feeling kinda weak today"*, or *"Oooooh, Girls night out for cocktials? I can't, it'll interfere with my meds..."*, or my favorite: *"An all-white party! Guurrrl bye! Not the way I'm bleeding! Chile, I'm over here flowin' like the Nile river!"*

It disappointed me as much as it did them, when I had to repeatedly decline their invitations. In fact, they were not the only ones anticipating my return to "full-swing" just in time for the summer. I thought I would be "good to go" by then myself. When I wasn't, I felt embarrassed, hurt, angry, and disappointed. It hurt even more when the invites became more-and-more scarce or when I would find out about certain events only after the pictures had been posted on social media – and I wasn't in any of them. For the most part, my friends were incredibly understanding, but sometimes they just didn't get the point.

Knowing they keep our best interests at heart, and wanting nothing more than to see us happy-and-enjoying ourselves, sometimes even with the best intentions, our friends can be a bit overbearing and pushy. When we have to turn down social outings, sometimes our friends have a tendency to retort with: *"C'mon girl, it'll do you good to get out of the house...You know you wanna go!...C'mon, we've been waiting for this all year! It won't be the same without you!"*

While we recognize that statements like that usually come from a place of love and inclusion, what we need for you to understand, dear friends, is that when you say things like that to us: it only magnifies our sense of guilt and discontent. More often than not, it is not that we don't want to go; rather, we are in so much excruciating pain, or bleeding so heavily that we are literally unable to move. Therefore, as much as we would love to, we simply cannot go with you right then. We need you to honor that and not take it personally. We need you to keep inviting us out, in spite of the many "no's", because that one time you think you're doing us a favor by not asking us, may be the one time we're actually able to – and might really need to go. In the event that one of those must-do weekends falls at a time when we are having an Endo flare, try mixing things up, and make it a girls night *in*! Some ideas to consider might be: renting your favorite movies, ordering some swanky take-out, mixing up a few *mocktails* and bring the party to us! Trust me, it will do wonders to lift our spirits by confirming that those in our inner circle still care and have not forgotten about us. Battling Endo, we spend so much time alone by default; we really do relish the opportunity to bask in the company of our girlfriends.

As much as we enjoy the opportunity to get out-and-about when we can, sometimes social outings can be abnormally exhaustive. Conversely, a little alone time is sometimes what we genuinely need. A confusing irony, I know, especially considering the fact that we spend so much time dealing with this alone from the onset. I spent the entire last paragraph telling you how the presence of a really good girlfriend is vital in helping us cope. So, it can be confusing at times and difficult to balance the delicate dance of friendship while trying to manage this disease. Unknowingly, the darts of miscommunication, resentment, assumptions of being shunned, and lack of understanding can be thrown both ways when good friends are caught in the middle of endometriosis. Much like the consequence of a romantic relationship, occasionally, friendships are lost in the fray.

It would stand to reason that many of our closest girlfriends wouldn't be our friends, if we didn't have many of the same things in common. Musical interests, life philosophies, favorite authors, and yes, our periods are commonalities. In fact, most women have experienced at least once, the "syncing up" of their monthly cycles with other women. Sometimes in an effort to be relatable, and to help us feel like we're not alone, our friends tend to make one of the biggest, most un-intentionally hurtful statements that one can make, such as: *"Yeah, girl, I get bad cramps too. I know how you feel…."*

Oh, if Endo was only as simple a matter as having *bad cramps.* While severe cramping can be one of the more recognizable symptoms of Endo, having *bad cramps* do not even begin to describe the unbearable torment we have to a face on a monthly basis. If you have never been unable to move, bled so heavily that it soaked through a bed mattress, or experienced: vomiting, nausea, headache, or pain so severe that only opiate-based medicines bring minimal relief, you have no idea how we feel.

As explained in the blogpost *"What NOT To Say To A Woman With Endometriosis"* (2013)

> Endometriosis is not cramps. It's not even "bad cramps". It's chronic pain caused by internal bleeding and inflammation. There are two types of endometriosis pain: tolerable and intolerable. It can't be solved with over the counter medication or a heating pad. It's not the same thing as cramps. When they have an endometriosis flare up, most women are unable to move at all. Comparing that to cramps is incredibly degrading. [47]

While we know it is not intentional, reducing our pain to *bad cramps* can often make us feel that you are downplaying, or even minimizing our experience. Kelle O'Connell says it best in the blogpost, "Again, I understand the people who said these things had good intentions and were just trying to provide help in some way, but these words cut more than they heal." [48]

The same advice that I gave to the men, would apply here also. If you have a friend with Endometriosis, and you're not exactly sure what that means-educate yourself. Your friend may have tried to explain it to you only to leave you feeling more confusion than clarity. Just like the men in her life, you can accompany her to doctors' visits and informational forums as a means of solidarity and support. You can also join one of the many online social media groups open to friends of those with Endo. In addition, you can continue to be a sounding board by simply listening. You can take the challenge to step up when she needs a hand, or gently step away when she needs her space. In short, just continue to do the one thing, the most important thing that you've always done naturally: be her friend.

"What can you say....it's family" ~ Jill Scott.

On that eventful winter afternoon in 2009, as I was rushing to the hospital emergency room, not quite sure if it was my appendix or my intestines that were speculated to burst, my mother was the first person I called. When I groggily awoke from my first round of intravenous pain meds, my daddy's face was the first one I saw. Throughout that entire initial ordeal, my parents were right by my side: talking with the doctors, questioning the surgeons, and keeping me as comfortable as they possibly could. My Dad stayed with me for those critical first days after my hospital release and my Mom called every day to see if there was anything that I needed that she could bring to me. In the beginning, like me, my parents thought that once I had my surgery, my misfortune with endometriosis would be over; case closed.

So, when the symptoms reoccurred, the doctor's visits increased, and the relapses showed up, they didn't quite understand what was happening or even why. When I missed family get-togethers at Thanksgiving and Christmas – two years in a row – opting instead to have someone "bring me a plate" my mom was convinced I was trying to skirt my way out of making my family famous macaroni and cheese. One of her favorite questions to ask me concerning my pain was "Have you prayed on it?" Sometimes, before I could answer, she would just take over and start praying for me. I knew she meant well, but there were many-a-times that I sat there thinking: *"Mama, I love you to pieces, but I am all prayed out! I'm gon' start praying in tongues in a minute, cuz I'm fresh outta words to pray in English! Shoot, even Jesus wept! And right about now, I can thoroughly relate to his experience in the Garden of Gethsemane – for I often find myself crying out 'My God, My God, Why hast thou forsaken me!'"*

But that was my Mama. And prayer is Mama's answer for everything. I couldn't dare say anything like that to her – out loud anyway. Even though I would get tired of her asking, I must say, I am eternally grateful that she never got tired of praying for me (even when I was too discouraged to pray for myself).

There's an old adage that states: "If you don't have anything nice to say, then don't say anything at all." When trying to relate to a loved one with Endo, we know, more often than not, that it isn't that you don't have anything nice to say, you simply don't know what to say.

In doling out his special brand of wisdom, in the way that only he can, my Father has often told me, "Sometimes, it's alright *not* to have all the answers. It's okay to say, *I don't know.*" My father would quietly-and- patiently listen to me go on-and-on in my *ump-*

teenth Endo-rant, (as we sisters call them). When I'd finally uttered my last exasperated line, there were times when all he would be able to say is, *"I'm sorry honey. I wish there was something I could say to make it better."* Just saying that made it better. Simply having my pain acknowledged with a kind word and a gentle tone was enough.

He didn't judge me, he didn't belittle me, he didn't try to minimize, denigrate, or gloss over how I felt. He didn't berate me with a slew of "but's" or "at least's", for example: *"....but it could be worse" or "at least it's not..."* In contrast, I was thankful because he listened. While it is human nature to want to comfort our loved ones when they are hurting, if you ever find yourself at a loss for words when in the company of an Endo Woman, she may be more likely to appreciate you if you do not say any of these phrases highlighted in Living With Endometriosis' blog post (see below).

Figure 5:

> ## Nine Things
> ## You Should Not Say To A Woman With Endometriosis
>
> "Have you tried Ibuprofen?"
>
> "I mean, you look like you feel well so it can't be that bad."
>
> "You just want people to feel sorry for you."
>
> "If there isn't a cure, you're going to need to just toughen up and get over it."
>
> "It could be worse, at least you don't have cancer."
>
> "I knew a girl who had that and she was fine."
>
> "You're so lucky, I'd love to take that many days off of work."
>
> You just need a more positive attitude."
>
> "Yeah, I have cramps today too." [49]

If you are not quite sure of what you should say to a loved one with Endometriosis, at least be mindful of some of the things you shouldn't say. Supporting us in silence is a hell of a lot better than hurting us with sarcasm (even when said sarcasm is unintentional). Sometimes saying less, really does mean more.

CHAPTER 8
STAY IN THE FIGHT

"I'm still standing" ~Monica.

Relishing the success of my very first Endo Awareness event did not last very long. In earlier chapters, I relayed what had inspired me to move forward with the event: the news I had received during my third relapse, that my Endo had spread and was now threatening the remaining healthy parts of my reproductive system. Because I was so motivated to complete the task of putting together a great event, I pushed the weight of that news to the back of my mind; at least, until after the event was finished. And though no one would ever know it, through all the: speakers, photos, interviews, people saying *"thank-you"*, tears from inspired Endo Sisters, and praises of *"congratulations on a wonderful event"*, my effervescent smiles and cheery disposition graciously disguised the fact that I was battling an excruciating flare-up the entire time!

Though some of my giddiness had waned in the days following that awesome event I was resolved to stay focused. Since I was in the middle of, yet another wait and see cycle, I went right back into research mode. I tirelessly searched to find other options that would complement the doctor's latest plan for treatment. It was then that I remembered some advice given to me by my neighbor and his girlfriend: Marquese and Olivia. Both were really good friends, as well as my neighbors and they were quite familiar with my **Endo** struggles.

Initially, I had always known Marquese as the "marathon guy that lived down the hall from me." Every time I would see him, he would either be: on his way out to run or just coming back from a run. Sometimes I would see him sprinting past me on the lakefront trail, while I was putting in my best powerwalk.

Whenever I would see Olivia, or "Liv" as we called her, she would always be reminding me that we need to get together to chat about how "eating clean" and changing a few of my eating habits might be able to help ease some of my Endo symptoms. I knew what she was talking about and I was very familiar with the concept of raw/vegan eating. In fact, I had even dabbled with it in the past. Up until now, however, I wasn't trying to hear anything about giving up any of my favorite foods, least of all, my cheeses and sweets! Those were my two favorite indulgences to have on hand whenever, *"The Lil' Heffa"* as I'd affectionately nicknamed my Endo flares, decided to rear her ugly head!

However, it wasn't until this latest flare-up that I remembered that Marquese wasn't just an avid runner, but he was also a fitness coach and Raw Vegan Nutrition Specialist. In addition, both he and Liv had just launched their program, *"The Proper Physique"* – a program that, among other things, teaches you how to heal from within by using the foundational properties of a "plant-based" diet. The next time I caught Marquese coming in from his run, I explained my latest development to him, and I told him that I was now ready to explore "The Proper Physique" plan! I was ready to learn how to do-or-undo whatever I might be doing with food, that may be contributing to the rapid reoccurrence of these Endo episodes! I was wholeheartedly prepared to: eat, drink, *or not,* whatever it was that might have even the slightest chance of keeping my fallopian tube from rupturing and saving me from another major surgery.

At this point, I had already exhausted several different options – surgical, hormonal, medicinal – all with varying degrees of success. By now I figured it could not possibly hurt anything to at least try to make a few changes to my eating habits. It would be a few months before I followed up with my doctor; so, I thought *"what do I have to loose except maybe a few pounds?"* And while weight loss was not my primary goal, if it happened to be one the benefits of the program, then hey, I would take it!

During the next six weeks, I gained incredible knowledge about the difference between *acidic* and *alkaline* foods, and the different effects they can have on the body including: increasing-or-decreasing inflammation (which is one of the most prevalent causes of pain and discomfort with endometriosis regardless of bleeding). In addition to my Endo journal, I also kept a food/symptom journal, where I not only recorded what I ate, but I also kept track of: how I felt and whether my Endo symptoms increased, decreased, or just stayed the same. In addition, I also participated in a detox program, where we eliminated certain "suspect" foods from my diet and replaced them with healthier plant-based options. Over time, I was able to pin-point very specific foods that either triggered full blown flare-ups or caused my symptoms to spike. After gleaning this knowledge, I immediately eliminated those foods, and replaced them with new foods that I had discovered during this process. Being a lover of all-things-food, and being one who loves to cook, this entire process was much less painful than I had imagined. In fact, I fully enjoyed learning new ways to cook and to "un-cook" many of my favorites foods. Additionally, I kept an open mind toward trying new foods that I had never even known about in the past. By the time I realized I had gone nearly a month without any dairy, I did not even miss it from my diet! I had also become much more "green" in my eating by incorporating: juicing, green smoothies, and even a bit more raw/vegan options into my eating routine!

The best part about this whole process, was that I was now able to draw a direct correlation between the certain foods that I ate, and the subsequent aggravation of my symptoms. Knowing this, and knowing how to manage this, had made me feel even more empowered in working toward controlling this disease instead of letting it control me. By the end of my six weeks on this program, not only had my daily back pain and cramping dramatically decreased, but I hardly had any random spotting, and the dull nagging ache on the right side of my lower abdomen was practically non-existent. My endurance for physical activity skyrocketed! I was walking up to four miles and rocking out to my *Shawn T's "Hip-Hop Abs"* DVD's 4-5 days each week! [50] I had achieved more relief and more freedom from the bondage of this disease during that six week journey than I had since the time before my diagnosis.

I knew what I had reported by tracking everything in my journals. I knew what I had felt in my body: the improvement in stamina, the increased energy, the decreased amount of pain pills. However, there were times when I still wondered, *"Had any of this made any difference at all?"* I could not ignore what I was seeing in front of me and I refused to believe that the modifications in my diet and exercise had not contributed to these positive developments. My hope, against hope, was finally confirmed when I returned to the doctor in June and he told me: It appeared that *all* evidence of fluid and swelling in my fallopian tubes was gone, the lining of my uterus was "nice and thin", and I could stay on my suppressive birth control therapy. Best of all, he told me that, when the time came, that I could actually try to conceive naturally! I had heard him clearly, when he used the word "try" but still – the possibility was there- so, I yet praised God for that! Now, I would just need that husband to show up!

Ecstatic could not begin to describe what I was feeling in that moment. To hear that no surgery would be needed, at least for now, was the best news I could have ever prayed to hear! I continued to reap the benefits as I gradually adapted this new change of eating habits and exercise into a permanent lifestyle. Eventually, I returned to the doctor in October for my next follow up and I couldn't have been happier!

October 11, 2012

So, had my quarterly checkup…and the prognosis seems to be pretty good. I'm down to 10mg of the Elavil and save for some light spotting periodically, everything looks good! Tube (still) looks clear, lining(still) thin, and I can still stay with the continuous BC so NO period! If all stays well, I don't have to go back for another six months!

I am pretty sure that for most of you, having a six month stretch in-between doctor's visits is not that big of a deal. But for someone who had had to show up every 2-3 months, travel by bus (anywhere from downtown Chicago, to Evanston, to Skokie sometimes all in the same week), only to be explored/exploited like a human guinea pig for the past FOUR YEARS…not having to go for six consecutive months was nothing short of a Godsend!

Please Note: Was there any scientifically backed, irrefutable medical "evidence" to undoubtedly "prove" that these positive changes were absolutely, 100% attributable to the changes in my eating lifestyle? No, it was not signed off on by the FDA, but my doctor seemed to believe enough in the correlation to encourage me to continue on that path with his full support. As I am not a doctor myself, I cannot guarantee any claims of improvement for anyone other than myself based on my own experience. What I do know is that implementing these changes in my own life have resulted in a dramatic improvement of: frequency, duration, and intensity of my symptoms. Additionally, I have talked with numerous Endo Sisters in my advocacy efforts over the years, about how implementing diet/nutrition modifications seemed to offer beneficial outcomes for them as well. Again, every woman is different and not every treatment option will work for every woman in the same way. It is simply my goal to offer information and insight on a variety of options, from one Endo Sister to another.

So, what exactly does all this mean? Was my six month reprieve from: doctor's visits, exploratory treatment plans, and surgery scares a permanent indication that my fight with Endo was over? Absolutely not! Did it mean that I would never have a flare up or ever find myself balled up on a gurney in an ER waiting room? Not at all. Did it mean that I would never have to consider the possibility of having more surgeries or adding adoption to the list of my family planning choices? Not in the least! In fact, in the two years following, and even to this day I still have intermittent cycles of remission-and-reoccurrence with my flare-ups and symptoms. There are still times where I have to: take sick leave from work, decline holiday festivities, or politely turn down suitors who ask me out on dates.

What that moment meant, however, was that just because I had Endometriosis, Endo did not have to have me! It meant that I did not have to sit idly by to allow fate or how I would live my life to be dictated by people who: did not know me, did not value me, and had no personal stake in the quality of my future. In that moment, for the first time, I walked through an option that I had chosen by myself and for myself.

I was a first-hand witness to the positive effects and results that I had accomplished by changing my lifestyle. I had become educated through my own: up-close, personal, and unique experience with this disease. I now had first-hand experience: in my body, in my relationships, in my life. It was that experience that had allowed me to become educated in ways that could not be paralleled in textbooks or case studies. I had also become enlightened: the knowledge I gained throughout my initial Endo experience could not be alluded to in any pamphlet, brochure, or medical consultation. No doctor could have prepared me for the hellish depths of: longsuffering, mental, physical, and emotional anguish that I would have to endure. Additionally, no doctor could have equipped me with the tenacity, faith, and inner strength that I would need in order to overcome. Educated, and now enlightened, I had also become empowered. I had chosen an option for myself and I had a voice in my treatment and management of this disease. I did not have to be bullied by the "professionals" or "experts", or let their recommendations be forcefully shoved down my throat without protest or alternate recommendations. My ONLY options were NOT to be drugged or cut open. While surgeries and medicines had their place, they were also accompanied by: talk and massage therapies, diet and nutrition modifications, exercise, support groups, and prayer. I had become a fearless, focused, advocate for myself. And now, I was becoming a bold, determined advocate for the more than 176 million Endo Sisters worldwide who have been suffering and are in danger of the same fate!

That moment showed me just how much of a fighter I truly was. It let me know that my journey would never be over. In spite of everything that I had endured over the past 48 months, I was still here, still strong, and still standing. But the fight was not over and there was more work to be done. As long as Endometriosis exists, with limited treatment options, and without a cure the fight would continue. For as long as I am here, for as long as I have presence, for as long as I have a purpose, a breath, a voice in this life – I will remain in this fight. I will fight long. I will fight hard. I will fight fiercely! *Will you*?

If you are a woman recently diagnosed with Endo, or suspect that you might be, you may be wondering what to do next? What should your next steps be? Where do you even begin? When I was diagnosed, I had these exact same questions. I have been where you are, and can empathize with your anxiety, confusion, and frustration. As such, it is my hope that the following tips will provide you with a clear, concise roadmap that you will find helpful for getting started.

The first thing I would do is follow the premise that you may have noticed throughout this book. It is not only the mantra for my business, and my life, but it is also the blueprint for my Endo awareness efforts: Get Educated, Get Enlightened, Get Empowered! Educate yourself by learning as much as you can from as many reliable sources as you can about what Endo is and is *not.* Use the enlightenment of your knowledge to make informed and comprehensive decisions for yourself about what course(s) of action will work best for you, your family, your career, and your life! Use your empowered voice to speak up, to push back, and disagree. Do not be afraid! Do not be afraid to seek second (or third or fourth) opinions from multiple doctors! Do not be afraid to refuse medications, especially if you are not well versed on *all* of their potential outcomes and effects.

Do not take any one doctor's word as *law,* especially if anything they say: does not sit right with you, makes you uncomfortable, or goes against any convictions you may have – be it morally, spiritually, ethically, or otherwise. Seek out different specialists and get several points of view. Be sure to exhaust all of your options. Be assertive! Be vocal! Be an advocate for you!

Throughout your Endo journey, you may be faced with having to make countless choices that relate to your treatment and care. If you find yourself metaphorically seeing *red flags* and hearing internal sirens telling the tale of *proceed with caution,* then I strongly encourage you to take heed. Every woman's journey is a personal, intimate, and unique experience. You know your body better than anyone, and you should have an absolute say in the planning and protocol for your treatment and care.

You are an individual. Your Endo experience, while similar to others, will be uniquely inherent to who you are; your personality, your lifestyle and your relationships. It will fundamentally impact the goals, dreams, and desires you have for both your personal and professional life. Your treatment and care should be a direct reflection of that distinct, personal, individual experience!

In considering the many choices you will inevitably have to make as your navigate your battle with endometriosis, there is one choice, in my opinion that should be considered above all others. More than the doctors, more than the treatments, more than the family planning options, the most important consideration should be **you**; what you need, what you want, how you will be affected. No one knows better than you what it is like to walk in the shoes of an Endo Woman. In the midst of all the: opinions, suggestions, perspectives, and choices I urge you, admonish you, encourage you…to choose **YOU** – All the time. Every time!

Until a cure is found and Endometriosis is eradicated from the lives of every woman, teen, and young girl currently suffering, we must continue to fight! We must fight to educate the uninformed. We must fight to enlighten the unaware. We must fight to empower our fellow Endo Sisters , so they do not get lost in the fray! We must fight boldly. We must fight continuously. We must fight… FIERCELY!

EPILOUGE

Saturday (date unknown)

I know it sounds crazy, but somehow –even in the midst of all this madness- God is still managing[to keep me]. Somehow I know I'm gonna get outta this okay! Through all the fear, the doubt, the uncertainty – somewhere in me and somewhere in all of this – I know...

"It doesn't matter what they say or do, don't let 'em get to you. Don't be afraid You can, you can, you can breakthrough! Take what I've been through, to see that, you can't hold a good woman down. Went through the same point of givin' up, felt like I had enough, went to the edge of the ledge, but I didn't jump - my life will sum it up - you can't hold a good woman down" *~Mary J. Blige, Good Woman Down.*

APPENDIX

Common Myths about Endometriosis

Endometriosis Support Groups and Organizations

Doctors Specializing in Treatment of Endometriosis

Complementary Practitioners

Glossary of Terms

Notes

COMMON MYTHS ABOUT ENDO

There are a number of prevalent myths regarding Endometriosis that are still being touted as facts to varying degrees. During my own Endo journey, I've had quite a few options suggested to me based on these myths. Many times, it was insisted that I could cure my Endo or prevent it from reoccurring.

A great place to start when evaluating what the next step(s) should be in your Endo journey, might be to investigate some of the most common myths surrounding it. Knowing what's true and not true can help provide clarity and direction when sorting through all of your options. The last thing you want to do is make a decision based on an unfounded myth and end up with long term or even permanent consequences that you find yourself regretting. You should never make a decision based on myths or faulty information.

Though by no means an exhaustive list, here are some of the more common myths to be mindful of when deciding how you should proceed in your treatment planning:

ENDOMETRIOSIS CAN BE CURED

"There is currently no absolute cure for Endometriosis, but there are several methods of treatment, which may alleviate some of the pain and symptoms associated with it." [51]

It wasn't until after I had my surgery that I was informed of the fact that there was no definitive cure for Endo. Had I known this going in, it most certainly would have had an impact on my decision to consent to certain forms of hormonal treatment options, namely *Lupron*. For many women, it provides great benefits in helping them manage their symptoms. For me, it did not. Had I known upfront that there was no cure for Endo, then I would have never allowed myself to be subjected to the horrendous side effects caused by *Lupron* in exchange for the miniscule amount of relief it provided.

GETTING PREGNANT CURES ENDOMETRIOSIS

Endometroisis.org states: "No. Some women find that their pain symptoms are reduced during pregnancy, but this is not the case for everyone. In most cases, endometriosis will return after giving birth and stopping breast feeding." [52]

The Endometriosis Research Center (ERC) also adds: "Only you and your partner know whether it's the right time in your life to become parents. Pregnancy should never be prescribed as a treatment for an illness! Pregnancy can keep symptoms at bay for some women, but it is not a cure." [53]

I cannot count the number of times that I wished members of the ERC were standing alongside me every time a doctor said to me: *"...Now, all we have to do is get you pregnant.";* As if getting pregnant would somehow automatically end all of my "Endo-woes."

With Endometriosis being "one of the top three causes of female infertility...", the ability to conceive is one of the foremost challenges faced by Endo Women.[54] Those who do conceive often report multiple miscarriages, and exhaustive physical difficulties, even when carrying to term. After delivery, many moms lament in our support groups about the dichotomy of finally becoming a mother, yet feeling unable to care for their newborns due to the belligerent resurgence of their symptoms. In talking with several of my Endo Sisters, I've found that getting pregnant is far from a cure for Endo. For many, it is literally *a labor of love.*

HYSTERECTOMY CURES ENDOMETRIOSIS

Dr. Andrew S. Cook, internationally renowned Endometriosis specialist and Founder/Medical Director of the **Vital Health Institute** recently remarked: 'The statement that you cannot have Endo after a hysterectomy is scientifically wrong, period. It is well proven Endo can and does persist, even after hysterectomy, both with leaving the ovaries in and taking them out. Endometriosis can produce its own endometriosis even without ovaries it has been shown in studies that endometriosis can have aromatase enzyme activity. Aromatase enzyme makes estrogen. [55]

Recently retired after 35 years of specializing in Laparoscopic Excision of Endometriosis, expert surgeon, Dr. David Redwine, added to Dr. Cooks sentiment by explaining on his website **Endopaedia:**

> "It is important to keep in mind, though, that not all pelvic pain is necessarily due to endometriosis. Some of the pain which may be relieved by hysterectomy/castration might have been due to problems with the uterus or ovaries, not due to Endometriosis. Therefore, hysterectomy/castration for 'Endometriosis pain' seems better than it really is. This helps to artificially magnify the apparent benefit of this procedure in the eyes of busy surgeons, who view it as a very effective and helpful procedure. However, this may be viewing the response of symptoms rather than the response of the disease." [56]

Since no one was able to guarantee, with absolute certainty, that getting a hysterectomy would definitively result in termination of the disease, and the cessation of all my symptoms, choosing this options was not a risk I was willing to take. Having read a number of   heartbreaking, regret filled stories of women who had received hysterectomies, only to have their symptoms resurface weeks or months later, solidified, at least for me, the fact that this course of treatment was not a viable option for me; especially since it was not a cure. To be clear, I am not taking a stance against hysterectomies. As with *Lupron* and other treatments that did not work in my favor, hundreds of women have gotten hysterectomies and experienced sustained relief from their symptoms. I tend to agree with Dr. Redwine's perspective regarding hysterectomies as further explained on **Endopaedia,** when he says:

> "Am I against hysterectomy or surgeons performing them? Of course not. It is a very useful procedure for uterine problems which do not respond to conservative treatments...However, I try to reserve hysterectomy for patients with symptoms suggesting that the uterus is a problem, such as **adenomyosis.** Although it may be successful in relieving symptoms, performing a hysterectomy with the idea of curing endometriosis is not scientifically sound, particularly if no attempt has been made to remove the endometriosis completely." [57]

On many occasions throughout my Endo experience, several doctors tried to aggressively force getting a hysterectomy on me as a means of providing long-term sustainable relief for my symptoms, despite my adamant objections. It was one of the most frustrating aspects of my battle. It was also one of the *fiercest fights* I ever had to face, knowing that first, this was not a cure for my disease, and second, this would completely obliterate my future plans of wanting to start a family. Nevertheless, I stood my ground with sure footed determination, and I refused to back down. *Fighting Fiercely,* score 1, hysterectomy, score 0.

TEENS ARE TOO YOUNG TO HAVE ENDOMETRIOSIS

According to **endometriosis.org,** " Far too many doctors still believe that endometriosis is rare in teenagers and young women... Consequently, they do not consider a diagnosis of endometriosis when teenagers and young women come to them complaining of symptoms like period pain, pelvic pain and painful intercourse... Teenagers and young women in their early 20s are not too young to have endometriosis – in fact, most women experience symptoms during adolescence, but unfortunately don't get diagnosed and treated until they are in their 20s or 30s." [58]

I was diagnosed with Endometriosis at the age of 33. I was subsequently told by my doctor's that mine was "...one of the worst cases they'd ever seen", and that based on the sizeable amount of disease that was found, their best estimate was that I'd had it for at *least* 10 years. However, based on my experiences described earlier in the prologue, I am now quite convinced that most, if not all of the symptoms I experienced throughout my teens and early 20's were almost certainly Endo related.

PERIOD PAIN IS 'NORMAL'

"'*Women's problems*' perplexed nineteenth century doctors, who saw them as indicative of women's unstable and delicate psychological constitutions... As a result, while seeking help for their pelvic pain (which may occur apart from menses), many women with endometriosis are told that their (often severe) period pain is *'normal'*, *'part of being a woman'*, or *'in their head'*. Others are told that they have *'a low pain threshold'*, or are *'psychologically inadequate'*. The net is that if pain interferes with daily life (going to school/work, partaking in day-to-day activities) it is not normal." [59]

When I relapsed with my Endo symptoms for the second time, I was told emphatically and with great conviction, that what I was feeling was *"all in my head."* A less vigilant woman, or one that is new to her diagnosis, might be tempted to concede to the perceived **power differential** of the doctor/patient relationship, but endometriosis.org declares that:

" If pain interferes with your day-to-day life, please seek help and ask to be investigated to determine the cause of your pain." [60]

ENDOMETRIOSIS IS AN STD/STI

In chapter 7, I discussed how Endometriosis can significantly impact a couples sex life, primarily by the effect of hindering a woman's ability to follow through with the act itself. When trying to explain the perils of Endo to a significant other, one of the most immediate reactions is to automatically correlate the cause and symptoms of Endo to that of promiscuous sexual activity. This is simply not true.

The Endometriosis Research Center validates this by stating: "[Endometriosis] is not a disease which is "contracted" or "caused" by anything the patient did - nor is it contagious." [61]

Those stating otherwise, are likely confusing endometriosis with **endometritis** – an inflammation or irritation of the lining of the uterus typically caused by chlamydia or gonorrhea. [62]

HAVING AN ABORTION OR DOUCHING CAN CAUSE ENDO

Of the earliest myths surrounding Endo, two of the most prevalent were that having an abortion, and/or regular douching was a leading cause of Endometriosis. Even today, decades after this theory has been disproven, lots of women wallow in guilt, shame, and embarrassment, somehow believing that having Endometriosis is their "punishment" for getting an abortion. Endometriosis.org adamantly refutes this claim, as evidenced in their research that shows:

"There is no scientific evidence linking abortion or douching, and consequently developing endometriosis. In fact, regarding abortion, it has been shown that: "women with endometriosis had fewer prior pregnancies, elective abortions, and ectopic pregnancies compared to women seeking care for infertility, who did not have endometriosis and …a reduced risk of endometriosis in women [who] reported a history of induced abortion has been reported." [63]

[Again], those who claim otherwise may be confusing "endometriosis" with *endometritis.* It is not the same as endometriosis. It is typically caused by infections such as chlamydia, gonorrhea, tuberculosis, or mixtures of normal vaginal bacteria and is more likely to occur after miscarriage or childbirth, especially after a long labor or caesarian section. [64]

ENDOMETRIOSIS ALWAYS LEADS TO INFERTILITY

The subject of fertility and endometriosis can be extremely confusing. On one hand, you have the evidence supporting the fact that Endo is one of the top three causes of infertility in women. On the other, you have members of the medical community presuming that all it takes is one good pregnancy to help alleviate your most harrowing Endo symptoms. Add to that the prevalent, yet permanent option of trying to attain relief via hysterectomy. It truly is enough to boggle the mind. However, research conducted by endometriosis.org, helps sort it all out by disclosing that:

"It is important to remember that having endometriosis does not automatically mean that you will never have children. Rather, it means that you may have more problems in getting pregnant.

Many women with endometriosis have children without difficulty, and many others become pregnant eventually — though it may take time, and may require the help of surgery or assisted reproductive technologies or both. [65]

It is estimated that 30-40% of women with endometriosis may have difficulties in becoming pregnant. This, however, means that 60-70% will have no problems. [66]

ENDOMETRIOS IS/CAUSES CANCER

The debate over whether or not Endometriosis is a form of cancer or if it causes other forms of cancer is a hotly contested one. In your own research, you may find that both lay persons, as well as "professional" or "informational" sources will refer to Endo as a type of cancer. Though many symptoms of Endo mimic those of other existing types of cancer, it is important to know exactly where to draw the line in the distinction between the two.

Women's Health (UK) indicates that: "Endometriosis is often compared to cancers that affect the female reproductive system, such as ovarian cancer and uterine cancer. This is because both endometriosis and reproductive cancers are characterized by cell invasion and abnormal cell growths. However, endometriosis is not cancer, and the growths associated with endometriosis are benign."[67]

Furthermore, *endometriosis.org* chimes in that "In very rare cases, endometriotic implants has led to cancer, but this is very very rare. Some research suggests that some women with endometriosis may be at a slightly higher risk of developing certain cancers but this is still controversial." [68]

In short, although similarities do exist between Endometriosis and cancers that affect the reproductive system, it has not been expressly established that Endometriosis causes, or is itself a categorical form of cancer.

ENDOMTRIOSIS IS ALL IN YOUR HEAD

In the book, *Endometriosis for Dummies* (2007) By Joseph Krotec, MD, and Sharon Perkins, RN , they explain:

"Even doctors used to believe that endometriosis was a psychological disease. The prevailing attitude was that, if you just stopped thinking about yourself all the time, all the pain would disappear. Some doctors actually believed that a woman's positive attitude would make the pain go away. Unfortunately, some professionals still use this rationale today. Although a positive attitude is certainly good to have throughout your life, you probably know that attitude doesn't decrease your endometriosis one bit. Endometriosis isn't just in your head (although it can be; endometriosis has been found in the brain! See Chapter 6 for more info) — it's in your pelvis, and it hurts." [69]

Let me be honest. In my experience, the absolute truth of the matter is, at some point while contending with endometriosis, you are going to have days that suck! You are going to have days where you are in a *funk*, when you can't be or don't want to be bothered. And you know what, that is perfectly okay. A long time ago, I developed a mantra to help get me through those kinds of times; especially when it comes to Endo: *"Feel what you need to feel, for however long you need to feel it, without explanation or justification to anybody."* You are entitled to your feelings; no matter how bad, how uncomfortable, or how *suck-tas-tic* they may be. No matter how awful the Endo cards you may be dealt are on any given day, don't let anyone guilt, shame, or *should* you into thinking that what you are feeling is all in your head.

ENDOMETRIOSIS SUPPORT GROUPS AND ORGANIZATIONS

There are a number of diverse support groups and organizations dedicated to the education, support, research, exceptional patient care, advocacy, and awareness efforts surrounding endometriosis. These organizations offer a wealth of medical, educational, and supplemental information designed to help you sanely navigate the often cumbersome, complicated, and confusing road a woman is likely to travel when dealing with Endometriosis. These are just a few support groups, informational websites, and organizations that I have found to be especially beneficial for me. I hope they are for you as well.

Online Support Groups/Forums for Endo Women, Friends, Family, and Loved ones.

Endometriosis Comprehension and support
An online community whose goal is to provide facts and treatment options that are available. Helping widen the knowledge of Endo sufferer and their supporters.
http://www.facebook.com/EndoComprehension

Endometriosis – A Family Affair
This page has been developed with the specific purpose of ensuring access to information, support, guidance, ideas and resources that may assist mothers, daughters, sisters, aunts, grandmothers, brothers, partners, fathers and friends who either have or know a loved one who suffers from Endometriosis.
http://www.facebook.com/pages/ENDOMETRIOSIS-A-FAMILY-AFFAIR

Endo Men – support group for husbands and boyfriends of women with Endometriosis
https://www.facebook.com/groups/273342296060619/

Endometriosis Couples – online forum to help men who are dating, engaged, or married to women with endometriosis (open to men and women)
https://www.facebook.com/groups/Endorelationships/

Friends and Family of Endometriosis Patients
https://www.facebook.com/groups/friendsandfamilyendo/

Mommy's with Endometriosis – for Mom's to be and caregivers with Endometriosis would have a safe place to come to talk about all things Endo related and their children without the worries of upsetting our fellow Endo sisters who are struggling to conceive or who can't conceive
https://www.facebook.com/groups/348039595235446/

EndoCenter of Chicagoland – a local branch of the Endometriosis Research Center and it is open to all women in the Chicago area including Chicago, the surrounding suburbs, etc.
https://www.facebook.com/groups/endocenterofchicagoland/

EndoMetropolis - Anyone who has an interest in the disease endometriosis is welcome (whether you are a patient, a professional or simply an interested on-looker).
https://www.facebook.com/groups/endometropolis/

Endo Warriors - a support organization for women who are focused on helping each other to fight against the devastating effects of endometriosis
https://www.facebook.com/groups/endowarriors/

Informational Websites

Endo Resolved - Advice and support to give you motivation, confidence and hope that you can restore your health and start to heal from the disabling disease of endometriosis.
www.endo-resolved.com

Endometriosis: A Guide for Teens
(offered by) Center for Young Women's Health
http://www.youngwomenshealth.org

Endometriosis.org – a global forum for news and information
www.endometriosis.org

Endopædia - is a comprehensive, online resource on the origin, diagnosis, and optimal management of endometriosis
www.endopaedia.info/index.html

Living With Endometriosis – Informational BlogSpot
http://www.livingwithendometriosis.org/

Teen Health - Endometriosis
http://kidshealth.org/teen/sexual_health/girls/endometriosis.html

Worldwide EndoMarch – global forum spearheaded by the Nezhat Family designed to empower, educate, and effect for the awareness of endometriosis via their 1st National Endo March on Washington in 2014. Get updates and information on upcoming Endo Marches.
www.endomarch.org

Endometriosis Organizations

The Center For Endometriosis Care
1140 Hammond Drive, Bldg. F, Suite 6220
Atlanta, GA 30328
Toll Free: 866-733-5540 Outside U.S.: 770-913-0001
www.centerforendo.com

The Endometriosis Association
International Headquarters
8585 N. 76th Place
Milwaukee, WI 53223
endo@EndmometriosisAssn.org
www.EndometriosisAssn.org

Endometriosis Foundation of America
90 Park Avenue, 17th Floor
New York, NY 10016
212.988.4160
www.endofound.org

Endometriosis Research Center (ERC) - ERC World Headquarters:
630 Ibis Drive
Delray Beach, FL 33444
Toll free (800) 239-7280 Direct (561) 274-7442
www.endocenter.org

DOCTORS SPECIALIZING IN THE TREATMENT OF ENDOMETRIOSIS

One of the most exhaustive aspects of my Endo journey was being bounced around from doctor to doctor, many of whom had very limited knowledge of endometriosis beyond a very generalized overview. It took me two years of back and forth, before doctors finally admitted to me that they had exhausted their scope of knowledge with regard to treating me and that they *"didn't know what else to do with me."* Had I been working with an Endo specialist from the beginning, I honestly believe that I would not have had as difficult a time as I did early on.

Since pouring myself into the Endo community over the years, aligning myself with various organizations and support groups, connecting with Endo sisters from all over the world, I have gained a wealth of knowledge about wonderful practitioners who specialize in the treatment of endometriosis, and many of the subsequent health issues that often accompany it. In fact, it was through one of my online support groups that I actually gained a referral to the specialist that I'm currently seeing now! Had I been able to work with him from the beginning, I'm absolutely convinced that my experience would have been much different.

If you are looking for a specialist in your area, both the Endometriosis Association and the Endometriosis Research Center are great resources for physician information and contact lists. Below are the names of a few specialists who have been known to have great outcomes in working with endometriosis patients. They have also been known to treat their patients with kindness, compassion, and vested interest in the best possible outcomes for the overall, long-term goals of their patients.

Please Note: The resources provided in this section is for informational purposes only. I do not personally attest to the depth or level of endometriosis knowledge that these practitioners may have, their level of skill nor, expertise, or their hospitality regarding patient interaction. These are practitioners that have been recommended for Endo Sisters by Endo Sisters. I cannot stress enough how important it is to remember that every woman's experience will be different. A positive practitioner experience for one woman many not necessarily result in that same experience with another woman. Conversely, a negative practitioner experience by one woman does not have to result in a negative experience for you. Even if you choose a completely different specialist, aside from the ones mentioned here, this list can still be a great resource for direction, clarity, and guidance in helping you sort out your options

California
Dr. Andrew S. Cook, MD, Founder and Medical Director*
Vital Health Institute
14830 Los Gatos Blvd., Suite 300,
Los Gatos, CA 95032
www.vitalhealth.com
408. 358.2511 or 888. 256.7705

Camran Nezhat, MD, FACOG, FACS*
Founder and Sponsor of Worldwide EndoMarch
Specializing in Multi-Organ Reconstructive Surgery
for Endometriosis, Fibroids and Infertility
Stanford Hospital & Clinics
900 Welch Road, Suite 403
Palo Alto, California 94304
www.nezhat.org/index.php
650.327.8778

Georgia
Dr. Ken Sinervo, MD, MSc, FRCSC, ACGE*
Medical Director
Center For Endometriosis Care
1140 Hammond Drive - Perimeter Town Center
Building F - #6220
Atlanta, GA 30328
www.centerforendo.com
866.733.5540

Illinois
Dr. Frank Tu, MD, MPH
Northshore Medical Group
Department of Obstetrics and Gynecology
Director, Gynecological Pain and Minimally Invasive Surgery

Skokie Hospital
9600 Gross Point Road
Skokie IL 60076

Highland Park Hospital
777 Park Avenue West
Highland Park, IL 60035

www.northshore.org
847.926.6544

Ranae Yockey, MD – OBGYN
Advanced Women's Care Center
800 Biesterfield Rd Suite 750
Elk Grove Village, IL 60007
www.advancedwomenscarecenter.com
847.981.3698

Oregon
Dr. David B. Redwine (Ret.), MD,FACOG*
www.endopaedia.info

Texas
Dr. John F. Dulemba, M.D., FACOG
Gynecology; Pelvic Pain & Endometriosis
The Women's Centre
3321 Unicorn Lake Blvd,Ste. 121
Denton, Texas 76210
www.womenscentre.net
940.387.624

Wisconsin
Dr. Charles H. Koh, MD, FACOG, FRCOG
Gynecology, Reproductive Surgery & Pelvic Reconstructive Surgery

Columbia Saint Mary's Hospital Milwaukee
2301 North Lake Drive
Milwaukee, WI 53211

The Reproductive Specialty Center
2350 N. Lake Drive, Suite 504,
Water Tower Medical Commons Building
Milwaukee, WI 53211
www.reproductivecenter.com

*In addition to the information listed here, these practitioners also have fan pages and are active participants in many of the online support groups and forums on Facebook.

COMPLEMENTARY PRACTITIONERS

This resource list is for practitioners who are not medical doctors, but their complementary (i.e alternative) forms of treatment/therapies have proven beneficial to many women in many areas of their Endo treatment, including pain management and fertility. Again, I do not make any claims or guarantees regarding the efficacy of these treatments, I only offer the information as a potential resource that may be of assistance to you.

Judith Florendo
Florendo Physical Therapy
600 North McClurg Court, Suite A312
Chicago, Illinois 60611
312.337.8840
www.florendopt.com
info@florendopt.com

Works extensively with patients having a wide variety of pelvic and related spinal problems that are often chronic or long standing in nature.

Melissa Lynum, Massage Therapist, Doula, Health Coach
Roots In Wellness
1647 N Clybourn Ave., Second Floor
Chicago, Illinois 60014
773. 313.3305
www.rootsinwellness.com

Specializes in therapeutic massage and bodywork techniques

addressing the position and health of the pelvic and abdominal organs, targeting symptoms in woman, such as painful or irregular menstruation, infertility, endometriosis, PMS, difficult menopause and uterus displacement.

Marquese Martin-Hayes, Raw Vegan Nutrition Specialist and Olivia Gomez, Cofounders
The Proper Physique
773. 809.5483
www.properphysique.com
info@properphysique.com

Individualized programs designed to help you love yourself through nutrition and well-being. Programs focus on will helping you detox your body, discover what works for you and strengthen your Spirit to maintain good health.

GLOSSARY OF TERMS

Add Back Therapy - Add–back therapy is a small amount of pro-gesterone, or a combination of estrogen and progesterone, usual-ly prescribed in conjunction with GnRH agonists. The goal of using GnRH agonists and add–back therapy is to stop the endometriosis from growing, protect your bones, and lower the side effects of hormonal therapy with GnRH agonists alone.[70]

Adenomyosis - ad·e·no·my·o·sis

A form of endometriosis characterized by the invasive, usually be-nign growth of tissue into smooth muscle such as the uterus. [71]

Chocolate Cyst - one having dark, syrupy contents, resulting from collection of hemosiderin(a granular brown substance composed of ferric oxide; left from the breakdown of hemoglobin)following local hemorrhage. [72]

Danazol - /dan·a·zol/ (dah´nah-zõl) - a synthetic androgen(A ste-roid, such as testosterone or androsterone, that controls the devel-opment and maintenance of masculine characteristics) that acts to suppress the output of gonadotropins(a hormonal substance that stimulates the function of the testes and the ovaries)from the pituitary, suppress ovarian hormone production, and directly block ovarian hormone receptors. It is prescribed in the treatment of en-dometriosis. [73]

Dilaudid - d-lôdd, A narcotic analgesic (trade name Dilaudid) used to treat moderate to severe pain. [74]

Endometrioma- en·do·me·tri·o·ma

A circumscribed (encircled) mass of endometrial tissue occurring outside the uterus in endometriosis. [75]

Endometriosis - \ˌen-dō-ˌmē-trē-ˈō-səs\

Endometriosis is a condition in which bits of the tissue similar to the lining of the uterus (endometrium) grow in other parts of the body.

Like the uterine lining, this tissue builds up and sheds in response to monthly hormonal cycles. However, there is no natural outlet for the blood discarded from these implants. Instead, it falls onto surrounding organs, causing swelling and inflammation. This repeated irritation leads to the development of scar tissue and adhesions in the area of the endometrial implants. [76]

Endometritis - /en·do·me·tri·tis/ An inflammation or irritation of the lining of the uterus (the endometrium). It is not the same as endometriosis. It is typically caused by infections such as chlamydia, gonorrhea, tuberculosis, or mixtures of normal vaginal bacteria and is more likely to occur after miscarriage or childbirth, especially after a long labor or caesarian section. [77]

Fentanyl - fen·ta·nyl , A narcotic analgesic used in combination with other drugs before, during, or following surgery and also for chronic pain management. [78]

GnRH (Gonadotropin-releasing hormone) agonists - hormonal therapy widely used to shrink endometriosis implants, which relieves pain.[79]

Hydrosalpinx - hī'drōsal'pingks

An abnormal condition of the fallopian tube in which it is cystically enlarged and filled with clear fluid.[80]

Laparoscopy - A surgical procedure used as the primary means of diagnosing endometriosis; also used to treat endometriosis. A lighted tube is inserted into the belly button through which the surgeon can view the inside of the abdomen. Instruments can be inserted into other small incisions to remove or destroy endometriosis.[81]

Lupron – The trademark name for the drug leuprolide acetate. Used to treat the symptoms associated with advanced prostate cancer. Is used alone or with other medication to treat endometriosis. [82]

Mefenamic acid /me·fe·nam·ic ac·id/ (mef'ah-nam´ik)

A nonsteroidal anti-inflammatory drug used to treat or prevent pain, inflammation, dysmenorrhea(the occurrence of painful cramps during menstruation) and vascular headache. [83]

Power Differential – A concept used to describe a relationship between two people who are not considered peers and thus hold different amounts of power within that relationship. This is often seen in professional relationships where a highly trained professional is advising or helping a person without the same level of knowledge in a given field. Examples would be: Lawyer/Client, Doctor/Client, Massage Therapist/Client, etc. [84]

Pre Menstrual Dysphoric Disorder – A severe premenstrual syndrome marked especially by depression, anxiety, cyclical mood shifts, and lethargy—abbreviation PMDD. [85]

Repliva 21/7 -This combination product contains a mineral (iron) along with 3 vitamins (vitamin C, vitamin B12, and folic acid). It is used to treat or prevent a lack of these nutrients which may occur in certain health conditions (e.g., anemia, pregnancy, poor diet, surgery recovery). [86]

NOTES

Chapter One:

1. Web MD (2015). "Your guide to Premenstrual Dysphoric Disorder (PMDD)." Retrieved from: http://www.webmd.com/women/pms/premenstrual-dysphoric-disorder

2. Davis, C. P. (2014). "What are normal hemoglobin values?" Medicinenet.com. Retrieved from: http://www.medicinenet.com/hemoglobin/page2.htm

Chapter Two:

3. Endometriosis.org: Global Forum for News and Information (2015). Retrieved from: http://endometriosis.org/
    According to the website, "Endometriosis.org is the global platform which links all stake holders in endometriosis - one of the most common causes of pelvic pain and infertility in women."

4. The Endometriosis Association: Together We Can Make a Difference (2014). Retrieved from: http://endometriosisassn.org/

5. "The History of Endometriosis" (2014). Retrieved from: http://www.wdxcyber.com/history-of-endometriosis.html

6. Endometriosis and Me (2014). "Celebrities with Endometriosis." Retrieved from: http://endometriosisandme.weebly.com/celebrities-with-endometriosis.html

7. Endometriosis Association (2014). "What is Endometriosis." Retrieved from: http://endometriosisassn.org/endo.html

8. Taken from the brochure "What is Endometriosis" (2010) by the Endometriosis Association.

9. Saint Michael Hospital (2012). "More Explanations on Chocolate Cyst (ENDOMENTRIOMA)." Retrieved from: http://www.mylifestyle360.com/st-michael-hospital/blog/more-explanations-chocolate-cystendomentrioma

10. Ballard, K.D., Lowton, K., and Wright, J.T. (2006). "What's the delay? A qualitative study of women's experiences of reaching a diagnosis of endometriosis." Retrieved from: http://endometriosis.org/news/research/why-the-diagnostic-delay/

11. U.S. National Library of Medicine (2011). "Fact sheet: Endometriosis." Retrieved from: http://www.ncbi.nlm.nih.gov/pubmedhealthPMH0016289/

12. Ibid.

13. Ibid.

14. Ibid.

15. Ibid.

16. Endometriosis.org: Global Forum for News and Information (2015). "Symptoms." Retrieved from: http://endometriosis.org/endometriosissymptoms/

17. Taken from the brochure "What is Endometriosis" (2010) by the Endometriosis Association.

18. Gallenberg, M. M.D. (2012). "Diseases and Conditions: Premenstrual Syndrome." Mayo Clinic. Retrieved from: http://www.mayoclinic.org/diseases-conditions/premenstrual-syndrome/expert-answers/pmdd/FAQ-20058315

19. Endometriosis.org: Global Forum for News and Information (2015). "Diagnosis." Retrieved from: http://endometriosis.org/endometriosis/diagnosis/

20. Ibid.

21. The Endometriosis Association (2007). "Endometriosis Information: Diagnosis." Retrieved from: http://www.ivf.com/endoassn.html

22. Endometriosis.org: Global Forum for News and Information (2015). "Diagnosis." Retrieved from: http://endometriosis.org/endometriosis/diagnosis/

23. Endometriosis Association: Together We Can Make a Difference. (2005). "Treatment Options." Retrieved from: http://endometriosisassn.org/treatment.html

24. "Pain Medication." (2008). Retrieved from: http://www.livingwithendometriosis.org/pain-medication/

25. Ibid.

26. Ibid.

27. Flinn, S.K., M.A. (2008). "Lupron®- What Does It Do To Women's Health?" Women's Health Activist Newsletter. National Women's Health Network: A Voice for Women, A Network for Change. Retrieved

from: https://nwhn.org/lupron%C2%AE-%E2%80%93-what-does-it-do-women%E2%80%99s-health

28. Medline Plus (2014). "Leuprolide Injection." American Society of Heath-System Pharmacist (ASHP). Retrieved from: http://www.nlm.nih.gov/medlineplus/druginfo/meds/a685040.html

29. Taken from the brochure "What is Endometriosis" (2010) by the Endometriosis Association.

30. Ibid.

Chapter Three:

31. Intuitive Surgical Inc. (2015). "Da Vinci ® Endometriosis Research/ Da Vinci ® Hysterectomy." Da Vinci Surgery. Retrieved from: http://www.davincisurgery.com/da-vinci-gynecology/da-vinci-procedures/endometriosis-resection.php

32. Ibid.

Chapter Six:

33. Shakespeare, Richard III (1.1.1).

34. Dictionary.com

35. Ibid.

36. Urbandictionary.com

Chapter Seven:

37. Dictionary.com

38. Ibid.

39. U.S. National Library of Medicine (2011). "Fact sheet: Endometriosis." Retrieved from: http://www.ncbi.nlm.nih.gov/pubmedhealth/PMH0016289/#i341.s5

40. Ibid.

41. Endometriosis Association (2010) "What Is Endometriosis?" Brochure.

42. Biesner, P. (2013). "23 Tips for Men on Supporting a Partner with Chronic Pain." The Good Men Project. Retrieved from: http://goodmenproject.com/featured-content/marriage-20-tips-for-men-on-supporting-a-partner-with-chronic-pain/

43. Ibid.

44. Ibid.

45. Ibid.

46. O'Connell, K. (2013). "For the Endo Girls: What NOT To Say to a Woman with Endo." Living with Endometriosis. Retrieved from: http://www.livingwithendometriosis.org/2014/04/03/what-not-to-say-to-a-woman-with-endometriosis/

47. Ibid.

48. Ibid.

49. Ibid.

Chapter Eight:

50. Shawn T's Hip Hop Abs. Beachbody®. Retrieved from: http://www.beachbody.com/product/fitness_programs/hip_hop_abs.do?code=SEMB_HHA_MSN&mr:referralID=a70ef301-9a25-11e4-ab7a-001b2166c62d

Appendix:

51. Endometriosis Research Center. Retrieved from: http://www.endocenter.org/

52. Endometriosis.org: Global Forum for News and Information (2015). "FAQS." Retrieved from: http://endometriosis.org/frequently-asked-questions-faq

53. Endometriosis Research Center. Retrieved from: http://www.endocenter.org/

54. National Institute of Child Health and Human Development (2002). "Endometriosis." Retrieved from: https://www.nichd.nih.gov/Pages/index.aspx

55. Retrieved from: www.facebook.com/AndrewCook on April 3rd, 2014, 6:18 am.

56. Redwine, Dr. D.B. (2013). Endopaedia. Retrieved from: http://endopaedia.info/treatment21.html

57. Ibid.

58. Endometriosis.org: Global Forum for News and Information (2015). Retrieved from: http://endometriosis.org/resources/articles/myths/

59. Ibid.

60. Ibid.

61. Endometriosis Research Center. Retrieved from: http://www.endocenter.org/endofaq.htm

62. Endometriosis.org: Global Forum for News and Information (2015). Retrieved from: http://endometriosis.org/glossary/

63. Endometriosis.org: Global Forum for News and Information (2015). Retrieved from: http://endometriosis.org/news/opinion/abortion-does-not-cause-endometriosis/

64. Endometriosis.org: Global Forum for News and Information (2015). Retrieved from: http://endometriosis.org/glossary/

65. Endometriosis.org: Global Forum for News and Information (2015). Retrieved from: http://endometriosis.org/endometriosis/infertility/

66. Endometriosis.org: Global Forum for News and Information (2015). Retrieved from: http://endometriosis.org/frequently-asked-questions-faq/

67. Women's Health: Health Information and More (2015). Retrieved from: http://www.womens-health.co.uk/cancer.html

68. Endometriosis.org: Global Forum for News and Information (2015). Retrieved from: http://endometriosis.org/frequently-asked-questions-faq/

69. Krotec, J. M.D., and Perkins, S. R.N. (2007). Endometriosis for Dummies. Hoboken, NJ: Wiley.

Glossary of Terms:

70. Retrieved from: http://www.youngwomenshealth.org/hormone-therapy.html

71. Retrieved from: www.medical-dictionary.thefreedictionary.com

72. Ibid.

73. Ibid.

74. Ibid.

75. Ibid.

76. Ibid.

77. Retrieved from: http://endometriosis.org/glossary/

78. Retrieved from: www.medical-dictionary.thefreedictionary.com

79. Retrieved from: http://www.webmd.com/women/endometriosis/gonadotropin-releasing-hormone-agonist-gnrh-a-therapy-for-endometriosis

80. Retrieved from: www.medical-dictionary.thefreedictionary.com

81. Retrieved from: http://endometriosis.org/glossary/

82. Retrieved from: www.medical-dictionary.thefreedictionary.com

83. Ibid.

84. Retrieved from: http://www.joylifetherapeutics.com/Pages/ArticlePower.php

85. Retrieved from: www.medical-dictionary.thefreedictionary.com

86. Retrieved from: http://www.webmd.com/drugs/

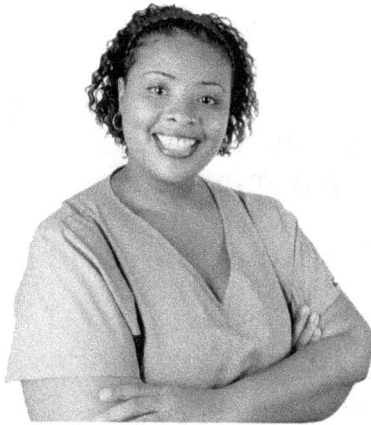

ABOUT THE AUTHOR

As a successful Licensed Massage Therapist and Wellness Educator, Michelle N. Johnson fights fiercely to educate, enlighten and empower individuals to become proactive participants in their health wellness management.

Blessed with a compassionate heart, and a strong desire for helping others, Michelle has always maintained a great interest in alternative therapies and the healing arts. After receiving her certification in Therapeutic Massage & Bodywork from The New School for Massage, Bodywork & Healing, (Chicago, IL.), in 2003, she went on to receive her Illinois State License in Massage Therapy the following year. In 2006, she become the President of her own therapeutic massage & wellness practice, Essential~E Therapeutic Massage & Bodywork, Inc.

Having been successful in the wellness industry for over a decade, Michelle passionately provides expert advice with honesty, integrity and sincerity. Michelle is an accomplished speaker, author, educator, wellness consultant, and passionate endometriosis advocate providing exceptional programs to individuals, small groups and corporate organizations. She brings annual awareness every March to the plight of those with Endometriosis with her Fighting Fiercely™ educational campaign. Michelle is licensed by the state of Illinois, and is an active member of Associated Bodywork and Massage Professionals (ABMP).

Michelle N. Johnson LMT, CIMI
Fighting Fiercely to Educate, Enlighten and Empower

"Michelle shares her endometriosis journey with honesty and sass! For those who don't have Endo, her story is heartbreaking—pain from the age of 11, and 20 years until diagnosis and treatment. Endo Sisters will simply nod their heads in recognition... Awareness of this chronic, painful hormonal and immune-system disease is key to early diagnosis and treatment. Thank you Michelle for your commitment to reach others so they don't suffer."

Carol Drury,
Associate Director/Education Coordinator
Endometriosis Association
www.EndometriosisAssn.org

If you would like to invite Michelle to educate, enlighten, and empower you at your next event, she can be reached at:

email:fightingfiercely@gmail.com

phone: 773.732.3163

Visit our website: www.fightingfiercely.com

www.ingramcontent.com/pod-product-compliance
Lightning Source LLC
Chambersburg PA
CBHW070922270326
41927CB00011B/2686